看護師のための
英会話ハンドブック
A Handbook of Practical English for Nurses

上鶴重美・Eric Skier 著

東京化学同人

まえがき

　ビジネスの国際化や観光政策の強化が進み,病院や診療所で働く看護師もさまざまな国籍の方々に対応する機会が増えてきました．グローバルなコミュニケーションに英語力は欠かせません．しかし,患者さんと意思の疎通を図らなくてはならない看護師の多くが,英会話に苦手意識をもっています．"患者さんに英語で話しかけられて返事に困った","簡単な説明でも英語の言いまわしがわからず慌てた"といった話もよく耳にします．嫌いなものや苦手なものは遠ざけておきたいという気持ちは人間の自然な防衛反応です．だからと言って"英語は苦手"と避けてばかりもいられないのが昨今の医療現場です．そこで少しでも皆さんのお役に立てばと願い本書を執筆しました．

　看護師向け英会話教材は書店でよく見かけますが,そのほとんどが看護師側の言い回しを中心としています．看護師が一方的に患者さんに何か言っているだけでは会話にはなりません．会話というのは双方向であり,言葉をキャッチボールすることで成立します．たとえば,看護師がこれから行う処置について患者さんに説明すると,返事や質問という形での言葉が患者さんからは返ってきます．それらを受けて看護師はさらに言葉を返す,というのが自然な会話です．会話と会話をつなぐちょっとした言葉遣いが特に重要で,共感や思いやりをそこに込めることもできます．本書ではさまざまな看護場面における会話を通して,自然な英会話と英語のコツを習得していただけるように工夫しています．携帯にも便利なポケットサイズですから,いつもお手元に置いていただければ幸いです．

　ところで,英語には日本語のような尊敬語や謙譲語という形での敬語はありませんが,丁寧語・丁寧表現があるという

ことをご存知でしたか？　日本語でも英語でも，患者さんやご家族に対応するときには丁寧な言葉遣いの方が好印象を与えます．しかしちょっと面倒なことに，英語では言いまわしによって丁寧さの程度が違ってきます．つまり，相手との関係性を考慮して丁寧表現を使い分ける必要があるのです．そこで本書では随所で丁寧さ順の表現方法を紹介しています．"知っている英語があまり丁寧な表現ではなかった"といった目からウロコの体験をしていただけるかと思います．

　英語を聞き取る力を鍛えて，伝わる発音を身につけ，英会話に自信をつけましょう．発音やリスニングは大人でも上達するそうです．自然な会話のリズムやイントネーションもご理解いただけるように，本書のすべての場面の会話をネイティブスピーカーが録音したCDを付録にしました．お手数ですが，とじこみ葉書でCDをご請求ください．すぐにお届けします．

　本書は，「薬学生・薬剤師のための英会話ハンドブック」（原 博, Eric M. Skier, 渡辺朋子 著, 東京化学同人刊）をお手本とさせていただいた姉妹本です．斬新な第一弾を企画・執筆・出版してくださった先生方に感謝申し上げます．今回は看護と英語，専門分野も職場も異なる二人の共同作業となりました．会話文は執筆者の経験に基づくものがほとんどですが，アイデアに詰まったときには多くの看護師の皆さんにご協力いただきました．本当にありがとうございました．

　最後に，本書の出版に御尽力いただいた株式会社東京化学同人編集部の住田六連氏および福富美保氏に厚く御礼申し上げます．

2011年1月

上鶴重美 (Shigemi Kamitsuru, RN, Ph.D.)
エリック M. スカイヤー (Eric M. Skier)

本書の特徴と使い方

■ **全般的な構成**：本書は，一般的な病院に勤務されている看護師の皆さんが使いやすいように考慮し，外来，一般病棟，周手術期，検査といった部署と状況で分けた5部構成にしました．第Ⅰ部は部署とは特に関係はなく，院内の至る場所でみられる何気ない看護師と患者さんのやり取りです．第Ⅱ部は"第1章 総合案内"から"第8章 救急外来"までの外来部門でよくある会話です．第Ⅲ部は"第9章 入院"から"第18章 退院"まで一般的な病棟で経験する会話です．第Ⅳ部は"第19章 手術前"から"第21章 手術後"までの周手術期を想定した会話です．最終の第Ⅴ部はさまざまな検査場面に必要な会話です．

■ **会 話 文**：一般的な病院で働く看護師が患者さんやそのご家族に対応するさまざまな場面を想定して，簡単なスキットにまとめています．話しやすい・伝わりやすいように，可能な限り**一文を短く**し，専門用語の使用はできるだけ避けました．英語表現は日本語表現を直訳したものではなく，**日常的で自然な表現**を紹介しています．

■ **Optional Phrases**：スキットの英語表現と一緒に覚えておきたい表現方法（**言い替え**）を紹介しています．表現方法によって丁寧さの程度が異なる場合は，**丁寧さの順番**がわかるように矢印を付けています．これを参考にして，できるだけ丁寧な英語を話すように心がけましょう．気分の悪さや厳しさの程度を紹介している箇所もあります．

■ **Additional Phrases**：スキットの英語表現と一緒に覚えておくと役立つ**関連表現**を紹介しています．

■ **Optional Vocabulary**: スキットの英単語と一緒に覚えておきたい**同義語**を紹介しています．

■ **Additional Vocabulary**: スキットの英単語と一緒に覚えておくと役立つ**関連語**を紹介しています．

■ **Eric's Tips**: **英語の特徴**, 英会話での留意事項, 外国と日本の**習慣や常識の違い**に関する助言です．

■ **Shigemi's Tips**: 外国籍の患者さんに対応する際の**看護師の視点**からの助言です．

■ **おぼえておきたい表現**: スキットの単語や文章と一緒に覚えておくと便利な英語を紹介しています．

■ **アイコンの説明**: 看：看護師, 患：患者, 家：患者の家族, 面：面会人, **OP**：Optional Phrases を参照という意味. 医：医学用語, 常：日常語, 男：男性語, 女：女性語, 幼：幼児語

■ **巻末付録**: 病院でよく使う説明用紙や記入用紙・様式の日本語版と英語版です．必要時コピーをとってご活用ください．

■ **索　引**: 病名, 症状, 医療器具, 応対でよく使う言い回しなどを五十音順に掲載しています．

■ **付録 CD**: 本書には, すべてのスキットを録音した CD が付いています．ネイティブスピーカーによる会話は, 最初のうちは聞き取りにくいかもしれませんが, 繰返し聴いているうちに耳が慣れてきます．リスニング力と発音を鍛えましょう．また自然な会話のリズムやイントネーションも真似てみましょう．

CD の発送について

　巻末のとじこみの葉書に必要事項をご記入のうえ，お送りください．折返し発送いたします．

■ **CD の内容**
　・12 cm　CD　1 枚
　・録音内容: Track No. 1〜67 のスキット
　・録音時間: 約 70 分
　・ナレーター: エリック　スカイヤー
　　　　　　　ワイスバーグ　エリカ

目　　次

本書の特徴と使い方 ·· v

第 I 部　は じ め に

Eric's Tips：英語での患者さんへの対応で大切なこと ············· 2

スモール・トーク ·· 5
　「ご出身はどこですか？」 ···························· Track 1 ··· 5
　　おぼえておきたい表現 **1** Yes, No のいろいろな言い方 ····· 6
　家 族 写 真 ···································· Track 2 ··· 7
　英 字 新 聞 ···································· Track 3 ··· 8
　天　　候 ① ···································· Track 4 ··· 9
　天　　候 ② ···································· Track 5 ··· 10
　日 本 語 ① ···································· Track 6 ··· 11
　日 本 語 ② ···································· Track 7 ··· 12

第 II 部　外　　　来

第 1 章　総合案内 ·· 14
　初診者への対応 ···································· Track 8 ··· 14
　受診科相談 ···································· Track 9 ··· 16
　車いすの手配 ···································· Track 10 ··· 18
　院内順路案内 ···································· Track 11 ··· 19
　　順路案内の表現例 ·· 20
　支払方法 / 会計の案内 ······················· Track 12 ··· 22
　面 会 受 付 ···································· Track 13 ··· 24

＊　Track 1 〜 67 までのスキットは付録 CD に収録されています．

第2章　診療科窓口 ……………………………………………26
受付・説明 ……………………………………… Track 14…26
呼び出し・計測 ………………………………… Track 15…28

第3章　問　　診 ………………………………………………31
問診・症状確認 ………………………………… Track 16…31

第4章　診　　察 ………………………………………………34
診 察 介 助 ……………………………………… Track 17…34

第5章　処　　置 ………………………………………………37
創　処　置 ……………………………………… Track 18…37
注　　射 ………………………………………… Track 19…40

第6章　診　察　後 ……………………………………………43
次回の外来診察予約・緊急時の連絡方法 ……… Track 20…43
処方箋と薬局 …………………………………… Track 21…46
診断書の発行 …………………………………… Track 22…48

第7章　入院手続き ……………………………………………49
入 院 案 内 ……………………………………… Track 23…49
個 室 料 金 ……………………………………… Track 24…51
入院時持ち物 …………………………………… Track 25…54

第8章　救 急 外 来 ……………………………………………56
救急患者への最初の確認 ……………………… Track 26…56
家族への説明 …………………………………… Track 27…58

第Ⅲ部　一　般　病　棟

第9章　入　　院 ………………………………………………62
自 己 紹 介 ……………………………………… Track 28…62
大部屋の案内 …………………………………… Track 29…64
病 棟 案 内 ……………………………………… Track 30…65

第10章　オリエンテーション ·· 67
　ベッド回りなど ·· Track 31 ··· 67
　電　　話 ··· Track 32 ··· 69
　食　　事 ··· Track 33 ··· 71
　　おぼえておきたい表現 **2** 年号, 日付, 時刻の読み方 ················ 73
　早朝検温 ··· Track 34 ··· 74
　午後の検温 ··· Track 35 ··· 76
　外 出 許 可 ··· Track 36 ··· 78

第11章　看護暦聴取 ·· 80
　面接の導入 ··· Track 37 ··· 80
　面接の終了 ··· Track 38 ··· 81

第12章　検査説明 ·· 83
　胃カメラ検査の説明 ·· Track 39 ··· 83
　心臓カテーテル検査の説明 ··· Track 40 ··· 86

第13章　治療・処置 ·· 88
　点滴の差替え ·· Track 41 ··· 88

第14章　服薬指導 ·· 90
　服薬指導 ·· Track 42 ··· 90

第15章　栄養指導 ·· 92
　栄養指導 ·· Track 43 ··· 92

第16章　離床・リハビリテーション ··· 95
　体位変換 ·· Track 44 ··· 95
　　おぼえておきたい表現 **3** 体の向き・位置・姿勢を変える ······ 97
　車いす移動 ··· Track 45 ··· 98

第17章　患者家族へ ·· 100
　家族の付添いについて ··· Track 46 ··· 100

第18章 退　　院 ……………………………………………………102
　退院準備………………………………………Track 47…102
　退院時の心配事………………………………Track 48…103

第Ⅳ部　周手術期

第19章　手術前 …………………………………………………106
　術前オリエンテーション……………………Track 49…106
　手術に必要なもの……………………………Track 50…108
　手術前の準備…………………………………Track 51…110
　　おぼえておきたい表現 **4** 頻度の表し方 ……………………112
　手術当日の準備………………………………Track 52…113
　手術室看護師の術前訪問……………………Track 53…115
　手術後の呼吸方法……………………………Track 54…117
　　おぼえておきたい表現 **5** ほめ言葉の程度 ……………………119

第20章　手術当日 ………………………………………………120
　手術室への移動………………………………Track 55…120
　手術室での会話………………………………Track 56…122
　手術中の家族への説明………………………Track 57…124

第21章　手術後 …………………………………………………126
　手術が終わって………………………………Track 58…126
　術後訪問………………………………………Track 59…128

第Ⅴ部　検　　査

第22章　検　　査 ………………………………………………132
　血液検査………………………………………Track 60…132
　尿検査…………………………………………Track 61…135
　　おぼえておきたい表現 **6** 分数の読み方 ………………………136
　血糖値検査……………………………………Track 62…136

胸部レントゲン線検査 ················· Track 63 ··· 138
CT 検 査 ····························· Track 64 ··· 140
上部消化管内視鏡検査 ················· Track 65 ··· 142
腰椎穿刺 ····························· Track 66 ··· 145
心 電 図 ····························· Track 67 ··· 147

付　　録

付録A　診察申込書 ································· 150
付録B　外来問診表 ································· 152
付録C　入院時の持ち物リスト ······················· 156
付録D　外出・外泊届 ······························· 158
付録E　胃カメラ検査問診表 ························· 160

索　引 ·· 163

Eric's Tips

1. 出身地には意味がない ································ 6
2. プライベート写真を勝手に見ないこと ················· 7
3. 6月のイメージの違い ································· 9
4. 天候が話題にのぼったら ····························· 10
5. 患者さんの気持ちを理解するために ··················· 15
6. 和製英語に注意 ····································· 19
7. 米国人はクレジットカードをどこでも使う ············· 22
8. サンキューにはサンキューでも OK ···················· 25
9. 前向きな表現を使いましょう ························· 29
10. 怒っているわけではない ···························· 33
11. 本当の男はお風呂が嫌い!? ·························· 38
12. 患者さんと何かするときはIよりもWe ················ 42
13. Meds は薬のこと ··································· 46
14. Hanko で通じます ·································· 50
15. 日本の安全神話の崩壊 ······························ 55

16. 名字の伝え方 ································· 63
17. 「ここは日本！」なんて言わないで ··················· 68
18. 複数形が一般的です ···························· 70
19. ワナ, ゴナ, ハフタ？ ···························· 72
20. "Pray"は慎重に使いましょう ······················ 84
21. 治療方針は誰が決めるのか？ ······················ 87
22. リハビリには愛のムチ ··························· 99
23. 質問には some も OK ·························· 103
24. 欧米の男性はストローを使わない？ ················ 109
25. 皮肉なジョークは聞き流しましょう ················· 112
26. 日本の医療に不安を抱く外国人もいる ·············· 116
27. 結婚指輪は外せない！ ·························· 121
28. ネバー・ギブ・アップ！ ·························· 129
29. 手順をふむときには First から ··················· 134
30. 「お疲れさま」は直訳しない ······················ 141
31. 患者さんはお客様？ ··························· 144

Shigemi's Tips

1. トイレは和式？ 洋式？ ·························· 66
2. "Stomach"で通じます ·························· 112
3. 百聞は一見にしかず ···························· 118
4. ゆるい指輪はテープで固定！ ······················ 121
5. 手術を待つ家族へのケア ························ 125

イラスト：望月さやか

I

はじめに

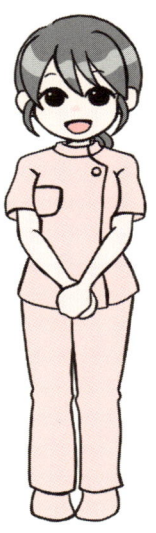

Eric's Tips
英語での患者さんへの対応で大切なこと

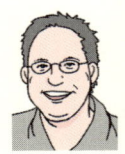

🔴 患者さんの目を見て話す
英語を話すときに一番大切なこと，それは，相手の目を見て話すことです．文法や発音をあまり気にする必要はありません．相手と同じスピードで話す必要も全くありません．

🔴 抑揚をつけて話す
二番目に大切なこと，それは，大きな声で，抑揚をつけて話すことです．質問をするときはいつも語尾を上げましょう．質問に答えるときや説明するときは，語尾を上げてはいけません．

🔴 丁寧な英語を使う
丁寧な英語(polite English)を使いましょう．覚えておきたい表現は，"please," "thank you," それと "excuse me," の三つです．このような表現を使って話すと，患者さんに良い印象を与えます．あなたの話し方は，あなたの印象になることを忘れないようにしましょう．

🔴 笑顔で対応する
患者さんには，できるだけ笑顔で対応しましょう．効果的なコミュニケーションは，言語だけではないのです．しかし，患者さんの言っていることが理解できないときは，決して笑ってはいけません．患者さんはあなたがなぜ笑っているのか理解できず，馬

鹿にされたと思って怒ってしまうかもしれません．

🔸 わからないことは調べて答える

患者さんの質問に答えられなかったときに，嘘をついたり，適当な情報でごまかしたりしてはいけません．また，日本語ではよく使う「まだ，わかりません」を，英語で"I don't know...."と表現すると「知りません」の意味になり，専門家として無責任な印象を与えます．"I can't say for sure, but....（はっきりしたことは言えませんが…）"とわからないことを認め，"I will look into it, and get back to you.（すぐに調べてお答えします）"と伝えて，適切な答えを準備しましょう．

🔸 患者さんにわかる言葉を使う

患者さんと話をするときは，専門用語ではなく，患者さんが理解できる簡単な言葉を使いましょう．また，できるだけ，短いセンテンスで話すようにしましょう．Simple is best !

🔸 主語には I よりも We を使う

患者さんへの指導やアドバイスの際，可能であれば，主語は"I（私）"よりも，"we（私たち）"の複数形を使いましょう．"I"がひとりの見解だと受け止められるのに対して，"we"だと組織全体の見解であるというニュアンスが出て，より信頼されやすくなります．

🔸 理解できないときは丁寧に聞き返す

患者さんから英語で話しかけられ，そのことが理解できなかったときに「エッ？」と日本語で返事をするのは止めましょう．"excuse me,"とか"pardon me,"または"I am sorry, could you repeat that？（すみません，もう一度言って頂けますか？）"と丁寧に言って，もう一度話してもらいましょう．

患者さんの考えを尊重する

異なる宗教をもつ患者さんは，健康管理についても異なった考えをもっています．個人の宗教や慣習・文化を尊重しましょう．

良いコミュニケーションは話し手がつくる

「お互いが理解するために誰が責任をもつか」という点で，日本と英語圏のコミュニケーションでは大きな違いがあります．英語圏においては，良いコミュニケーションを図るのは，常に話し手の責任です．

スモール・トークを活用する

患者さんと small talk（世間話）をしてみましょう．良い人間関係をつくるために，世間話が役立つことが知られています．慌ただしい医療の現場だからこそ，患者さんはホッとするような普通の会話を求めているかもしれません．

スモール・トーク
Small Talk

スモール・トークの例をいくつか紹介します．

「ご出身はどこですか？」
"Where are you from?"

Track 1

看	オルセンさん，少しお話を聞かせて頂いてもよろしいでしょうか？	Mr. Olsen, can I talk to you about something?
患	ええ，もちろん．	Yes, of course.
看	半年前からお仕事で日本に滞在されていると伺っていますが，ひとりでお住まいですか？	I heard you've been in Japan for the last six months on business. Are you living alone?
患	いいえ．アパートに，2人のルームメイトと一緒に住んでいます．	Nope*. I live in an apartment with two other people.
看	退院後，ルームメイトに助けてもらえそうですか？	Will one of your roommates be able to help you after you are released?
患	ええ，とってもいい人たちなので．	Sure, they are really nice people.
看	それは助かりますね．ところで，日本に来られる前はどちらにお住まいだったのですか？	I am happy to hear that. By the way, where were you living before you came to Japan?
患	アムステルダムです．	I was in Amsterdam.
看	では，オランダのご出身ですか？ (⇨ Eric's Tip 1)	Oh, so you are Dutch?

---

* nope は no のくだけた表現です（次ページ おぼえておきたい表現 1 参照）．

6　Ⅰ.はじめに

愚 いいえ．両親はオランダ人ですが，ニューヨークで働いているときに私は生まれたので，ニューヨーカーです．

No. My parents are Dutch, but when they were working in New York, I was born. I am a New Yorker*.

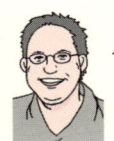

Eric's Tip 1　出身地には意味がない

日本では初対面の人に出身地(県)を聞くことがよくあります．しかし，欧米人に"Where are you from?"と質問した場合，出生地，育った場所，国籍など，さまざまな答えが返ってくる可能性があります．欧米人は出身地よりも民族性(ethnic background)の方をアイデンティティーとして重視しているようです．

おぼえておきたい表現
1 Yes, No のいろいろな言い方

"No"は，少し強い表現なので，あまり使いません．また，下表に示すように，否定の意味をもつ言葉には丁寧さに違いがあるので気をつけましょう．("Yes"には丁寧さの違いはありません．)

"Yes"の意味をもつ表現	対応する否定の表現	否定の表現の丁寧さ
No problem.	I'm afraid not. / I'm sorry, ...*	より丁寧 ↑ 丁寧さ
Sure.　Un huh.　Yep.　Absolutely.	Un un.　Nope.	

* 必ず後ろに断わりの理由を示す会話が続く．

---

* New Yorker という国籍はもちろんありませんが，ニューヨーク出身者はこのように冗談まじりに表現することがあります．

家族写真
Family Pictures

Track 2

看 マルコスさん,おはようございます.	Good morning, Mr. Marcos.
患 おはよう.	Hi.
看 どうなさいましたか?	What's wrong?
患 家族が恋しいのです.あるのはこの写真だけ.	I miss my family. All I have are these pictures.
看 拝見してもよろしいですか?(⇨ Eric's Tip 2)これはどなたですか?	May I have a look? Who's this?
患 妻のアンジェラです.	That's my wife, Angela.
看 おきれいな方ですね.奥様の隣の方は誰ですか?	She's very pretty. And who is next to her?
患 息子のカルロス.来週で5歳になります.	That's my son, Carlos. He's going to be five next week.
看 素敵なご家族ですね.見せて下さって,ありがとうございました.	You have a beautiful family. Thanks for sharing.
患 早く皆に会いたいです.	I can't wait to see them.
看 ご家族の皆さんも同じ気持ちだと思います.では,お食事のトレイを片づけてからお薬をお持ちしますね.	And I am sure they can't wait to see you! Now, let me take your tray and I'll be by in a little while with your meds.

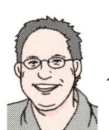

Eric's Tip 2　プライベート写真を勝手に見ないこと
外国人のなかには,プライベートな写真は誰にも見せたくないと思っている人もいるので,丁寧に許可を取ってから見せてもらうようにしましょう.

英字新聞
English Newspapers

患	看護師さん，すみません，ちょっといいですか？	Excuse me, nurse, can you help me?
看	はい，どうなさいましたか？	Sure. How can I be of help?
患	退屈で困っています．英字新聞はどこかで売っていますか？	I have so much free time and nothing to do. Are there any newspapers in English here?
看	下の階の売店に置いてあるかもしれません．電話して聞いてみましょうか？	I think the shop downstairs may have some. Would you like me to call and find out for you?
患	お願いできますか．そうして頂けると助かります．	Could you? That would be really great!
看	お気持ちはわかります．世の中のニュースを知りたいのではありませんか？	I understand your feelings. You must want to hear what's going on in the world, don't you?
患	そのとおり．こんなところにいたら，何が起きているのか全くわかりません．	That's right. Stuck here, I have no idea what's going on!

天候 ①
Weather ①

Track 4

看 ジェフさん，ご気分はいかがですか？	Hi, Jeff, how are you today?
患 まあまあです．でも，天気が良ければ，外に出て新鮮な空気を吸いたいところです．	I'm OK, but I wish the weather were nicer so I could go out and get some fresh air.
看 そうですね．でもこんな天気が普通ですよ．	I know what you mean, but this is actually quite normal.
患 6月はいつも雨が降っているのですか？（⇨ Eric's Tip 3）	Does it always rain so much in June?
看 そうです．日本で初めて経験される梅雨ですか？	That's right! This is your first rainy season in Japan, isn't it?
患 ええ，最低．	Yeah, and it sucks.
看 外に出たければ，傘を持ってきましょうか？	Well, I could get you an umbrella if you really want to go out.
患 お願いできますか？ そうして頂けると嬉しいです．	Could you? I would really appreciate that!

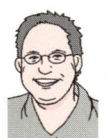

Eric's Tip 3　6月のイメージの違い
欧米人にとって6月は夏休みが始まり，初夏のよいイメージがあります．日本の6月は，休みもなく天気も悪く，ショックを受ける人が多いかもしれません．

天　候 ②
Weather ②

Track 5

患 雨が降っていても，外に出てみたいのです．	Even in this weather, I am happy to be outside.
看 一日中ずっと病室にいるのはつらいですね．	I am sure it must be tough staying inside all day long.
患 本当につらいです．	You have no idea!*
看 でも，梅雨はもうすぐ終わります．夏の東北はいいですよ．	But the rainy season will be over soon and summer in Tohoku is pretty nice.
患 友人もそう言っていました．でも，日本では秋が一番いい季節だと聞いています．あなたの好きな季節は？	That's what my friends say. But, they say that fall in Japan is their favorite season. How about you?
看 私は日本人ですから，好きなのは春です．桜の花とか．	I'm Japanese and can't help but love spring. It's a cherry blossom thing.
患 なるほど．ピンクや白や薄紫．きれいな花が咲くのでしょうね．	I see. Pink and white and purple. The blossoms are quite beautiful, aren't they?
看 それにお酒も楽しめます．「花見」と呼びます．	And we get to drink, too. It's called "hanami."
患 聞いたことがあります．楽しそうですね．	I heard about that. Sounds crazy!
看 楽しいですよ．	It's fun.

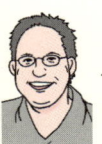

Eric's Tip 4　天候が話題にのぼったら…
何も話題のないとき，天候について話をするのが欧米人の常識です．つまり，欧米人があなたに話しかけ，天候を話題にしたら，「あなたと私には何も共通の話題がない」とほのめかしているのかも….

＊　患者さんはこのようにつらさを訴えることもあります．

日本語 ①
Nihongo ①

Track 6

看	こんにちは，サリカさん．何をなさっているのですか？	Hello, Sarica. What are you doing?
患	日本語の勉強です．	I'm studying Japanese.
看	えらいですね．見せて頂けますか？	Good for you! May I see?
患	これは漢字カードです．自分で作りました．	These are my kanji cards. I made them myself.
看	ええ，わかります．よくできていますね．テストしてみましょうか？	I can see that. These are really nice! Can I test you?
患	ええ．全部覚えていますよ．	Sure. I know them all!
看	さあ，どうでしょう．では，これは何？	We'll see. OK...what's this?
患	それは…言わないで．それは"鳥"．	That's...don't tell me! That's "tori."
看	ピンポーン．これは？	That's right! And this one?
患	それは"風"．	That's "kaze."
看	よく覚えましたね．退院するころには，たくさんの漢字を読めるようになりますね．	Very good! By the time you are ready to go home you'll be able to read a lot of kanji.
患	今月の目標は300字です．	My goal is 300 kanji characters this month.

日 本 語 ②
Nihongo ②

Track 7

患	すみません．看護師さん，これは何と書いてあるのですか？	Excuse me, nurse, how do I read this word?
看	それは私の職業の漢字です．"看護師"と書いてあります．	That's my kanji! It says, "kangoshi."
患	文字には意味があるのですか？	Do the characters have a meaning?
看	はい，あります．最初の二つは"ケア・面倒をみること"を意味しています．最後の文字は"専門家"を表しています．	Yes, they do. These two mean "care." And the last one means a "professional."
患	そのとおりですね．面倒見の良い人じゃないと，看護師にはなれませんね．	That makes sense! You have to be a caring person to be a nurse!
看	おっしゃるとおりです．	Exactly!
患	この単語はどうですか？	How about this word?
看	"sui-you-bi"と読みます．つまり，水曜日のことです．	That's "sui-you-bi." It means Wednesday.
患	sui-you-biですね．わかりました．ありがとう．	Sui-you-bi. I see. Thanks!
看	この調子で頑張って下さい．	Keep up the good work!
患	ありがとう．そうします．	Thanks, I will!

II

外　　来

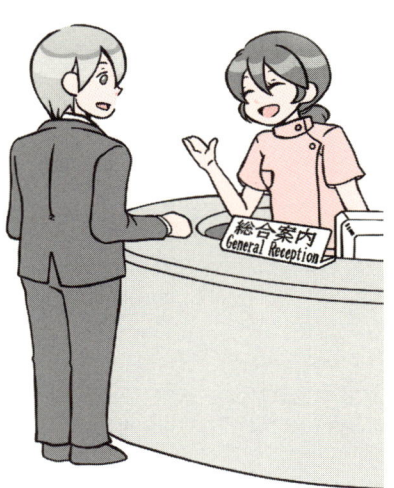

1

総合案内
General Reception Desk

以下の会話は一般職員の方々にも通用するでしょう．

初診者への対応
Attending to First-time Patients

Track 8

看	おはようございます．	Good morning.
患	受診したいのですが．(⇨ **OP**)	I would like to see a doctor.
看	こちらの病院は初めてですか？	Is this your first time to this clinic?
患	はい，そうです．	Yes, that's right.
看	紹介状をお持ちですか？	Do you have a letter of introduction from another doctor?
患	いいえ，持っていません．	No, I don't.
看	まず，この診察申込書（付録A, p.150）に必要事項をお書き下さい．	OK. First, please fill out this questionnaire.
患	はい，できました．	Here you go. I'm done.
看	では向かい側にある1番の新患受付（初診受付）に行き，診察申込書に保険証を添えてお出し下さい．カルテと診察券をお作りします．その後のご	Now, please go over by sign number 1 for new patients and be ready to present your paperwork with your health insurance card. They will take

案内は係員がいたします. your paperwork and make a chart and a patient ID card. After that someone will show you where to go.

患 わかりました.　　　　　　I see.

▶ Optional Vocabulary

初診者　first-time patient, new patient ／　紹介状　referral 医, letter of introduction 常, letter from your doctor 常, letter from a doctor 常, letter from another doctor 常, referral letter 医 ／　医師　doctor 常, physician 医 ／　看護師　nurse 常, RN (registered nurse) 医 *1 ／　患者　patient 常, client 医 *2

Optional Phrases

🔲 受診したいのですが.
　(⇨ Eric's Tip 5)

I insist on seeing a
　doctor!
I really need to see a
　doctor!
I need to see a doctor.
I would like to see a
　doctor.
Can I see a doctor?

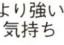より強い気持ち

強さ

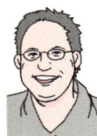

Eric's Tip 5　患者さんの気持ちを理解するために
"I need to see a doctor." の方が "I would like to see a doctor." よりも，患者さんの不安な気持ちが強く表れています．患者さんが緊急を要する事態であることを訴えていると解釈しましょう．

---

*1　RN: 登録看護師（日本の看護師に該当する．）
*2　client は，おもに外来などの通院施設において patient の同義語として使われます．提供される医療サービスが疾病治療のときよりも健康維持の場合に使われることが多いようです．

受診科相談
General Consultation

Track 9

患 あの…, ちょっとお聞きしてもいいですか?	Umm...can I ask you a question?
看 はい. どうなさいましたか?(⇨ OP)	Sure. **How can I be of help?**
患 2, 3日前から耳鳴りがするのですが, どの科を受診すればよいでしょうか.	About 2-3 days ago, I started having a ringing in my ear. Which department should I go to?
看 **ほかに何か症状はありますか?**(⇨ OP)	**Do you have any other symptoms?**
患 頭痛がします.	I also have a headache.
看 めまいはどうですか?	Do you feel dizzy at all?
患 めまいはしません.	Nope. I'm not dizzy.
看 血圧はどうですか?	How's your blood pressure?
患 最近, 健康診断を受けていないのでわかりません.	I don't know as I haven't had a check-up recently.
看 まず内科を受診して下さい. その後で, ほかの科を受診して頂くことになるかもしれません. まもなく係の者がご案内しますから, 少しお待ち下さい. (⇨ OP)	First, please go to internal medicine. After that, you may have to be seen in another department. In a moment, someone will show you where to go. **Please have a seat.**

▶ Optional Vocabulary

耳鳴り　ringing in my ear[常], buzzing in the ear [常], tinnitus[医] ／
めまい　dizziness[常], vertigo[医] ／　健康診断　check-up[常],
physical exam[常], health screening[医]

1. 総合案内　17

Optional Phrases

◘ どうなさいましたか？

How can I be of assistance?
How can I be of help?
May I help(you)?
Can I help(you)?
What's wrong?*¹
What's wrong with you?(失礼な表現)*¹

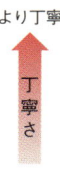
より丁寧
丁寧さ

◘ ほかに何か症状はありますか？

Do you have any other symptoms?
What other symptoms do you have?
What else is bothering you?

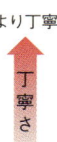
より丁寧
丁寧さ

◘ 少しお待ち下さい．

Please have a seat.*²
Please wait a moment.
Please wait a minute.
Please wait a second.
Please wait a sec.

より丁寧
丁寧さ

---

*¹ "What's wrong?"を使うときには表情とトーンに気をつけ，やさしい声と表情を心がけましょう．"What's wrong with you?"は「あんたの問題は何？」といった意味合いになってしまうので，使わない方がベターです．

*² 患者さんは病気なので"Please wait a moment."と言うよりも，"Please have a seat."として席を勧めた方が丁寧な対応になります．

車いすの手配
Arranging for a Wheelchair

Track 10

家 母を連れてきているのですが，足が悪いので車いすを貸して頂けますか？	I have my mother with me, but it's hard for her to walk. Can I borrow a wheelchair?
看 はい．玄関脇に置いてある車いすをお使い下さい（⇨ OP）．お手伝いが必要ですか？（⇨ OP）	Sure. **Please use one of the wheelchairs by the entrance. Do you need a hand**?
家 いいえ．たぶんひとりで大丈夫です．ありがとう．	No, I think I can manage on my own. Thanks.
看 必要であれば，いつでも声をかけて下さい．（⇨ OP）	**If need be, feel free to ask for help anytime.**
家 ありがとうございます．そうさせて頂きます．	Many thanks. I will be sure to do so.

Optional Phrases

○ 玄関脇に置いてある車いすをお使い下さい．

Please use one of the wheelchairs by the entrance.

Feel free to use one of the wheelchairs by the entrance.

You can use one of the wheelchairs by the entrance.

You can use a wheelchair from over there. （やや雑な表現）

○ お手伝いが必要ですか？

Do you need any assistance?

Do you need any help?

Do you need a hand?

Can you do it by yourself?（失礼な表現）

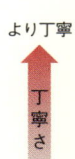

必要であれば，いつでも声をかけて下さい．	If necessary, feel free to ask for help anytime.
	If necessary, feel free to ask anytime.
	If need be, feel free to ask for help anytime.
	If need be, feel free to ask anytime.

院内順路案内
Giving Directions in the Hospital

Track 11

超音波検査室はどこでしょうか．	Excuse me, where is the ultrasound room?
地下1階です（⇨ Eric's Tip 6）．この先のエスカレーターをお使い下さい．降りてから右手に進むと，つき当たりが超音波検査室です．受付で予約票と診察券をお出し下さい．	It is on the first floor of the basement. Please use the escalator over there. When you get off the escalator, go to your right and you will see the ultrasound room. Please hand your appointment card and patient ID card to the person at the reception desk.
わかりました．ありがとうございます．	I see. Thank you very much.

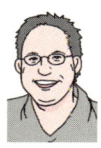

> **Eric's Tip 6　和製英語に注意**
> 日本では地下1階をB1と表現することが多いですが，B1は英語ではありません．正しい表現は the first floor of the basement です．ほかにもギプス（cast），レントゲン（X-ray），カルテ（chart），シャーカステン（display），エント（discharge），カルチ（cancer）などがあります．括弧内が正しい英語です．覚えておきましょう．

■ 順路案内の表現例 ■

ここでは，次ページの院内地図を例に，総合案内からの順路を示します．

① 内科へ

患 内科はどこでしょうか？ — Excuse me, where is internal medicine?

看 内科は廊下の突き当たりです． — It's at the end of the hall.

② 耳鼻咽喉科へ

患 耳鼻咽喉科にはどう行けばいいですか？ — Can you tell me how to get to the ear, nose, and throat doctor?

看 耳鼻咽喉科ですね．廊下を進んで左に曲がって下さい．外科の向かい側です． — The ear, nose, and throat doctor? Go down this hall and turn left. It will be across from the surgery department.

③ 車いす用トイレへ

患 車いす用トイレはありますか？ — Is there a wheelchair accessible toilet around here?

看 はい，右側の廊下を少し進むと右手にあります． — Go down the hallway on the right and it will be to the right.

④ エレベーターへ

患 エレベーターはどこでしょう？ — Excuse me, where can I find an elevator?

看 階段の先にあります．ご案内します． — You'll find one next to the stairs. Come with me and I'll show you.

⑤ 小児科へ

患 小児科に行きたいのですが．　　I want to go to pediatrics.

看 2階にお上がり下さい．右側の突き当たりが小児科です．　　Please go upstairs. You will find it at the end of the hall on your right.

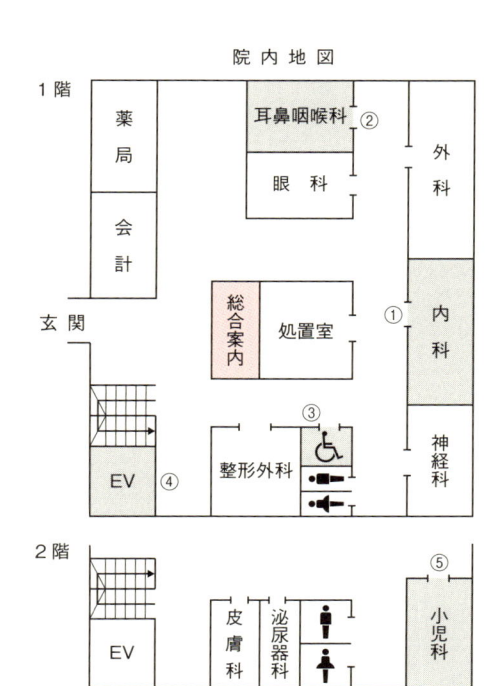

院内地図

1階
- 薬局
- 会計
- 耳鼻咽喉科 ②
- 眼科
- 外科
- 玄関
- 総合案内
- 処置室 ①
- 内科
- 神経科
- EV ④
- 整形外科 ③

2階
- EV
- 皮膚科
- 泌尿器科
- 小児科 ⑤

支払い方法／会計の案内
Giving Directions on How to Pay

Track 12

看	これで診察は終わりです（⇨ **OP**）．1階にある会計前の待合室でお待ち下さい．	**You are all set.** Please go to the waiting room in front of the cashier's counter on the first floor.
患	わかりました．支払いにはクレジットカードが使えますか？（⇨ Eric's Tip 7）	I see. May I pay with a credit card?
看	申しわけありません．お使い頂けません．現金払いです．	I am sorry, but you can't. We only accept cash.
患	現金をあまり持ってきませんでした．院内にATMはありますか？	I don't have much cash on me. Is there a bank machine in the hospital?
看	ここにはありませんが，向かい側のコンビニエンスストアの中にあります．	There isn't one here, but there is one in the convenience store across the street.
患	わかりました．行ってきます．	I understand. I will be right back.

▶ Optional Vocabulary

ATM automated teller machine 常, bank machine 常, cash machine 常／**クレジットカード** credit card 常, "plastic" 常(俗)

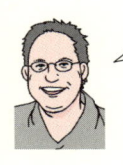

Eric's Tip 7　米国人はクレジットカードをどこでも使う
米国以外の先進諸国の多く（英国，カナダ，フランスなど）は，医療費の自己負担がないので，病院での支払いもないのが普通です．もしも患者さんが，"Do you accept plastic？"や"May I pay with a credit card？"と言ったら，たぶん米国人です．米国人はあまり現金を持ち歩きません．

Optional Phrases

◘ これで診察は終わりです。

We've done everything we needed to do.

We/You are done here today.

We/You are done here.

You are all set.

You are free to go.

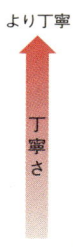

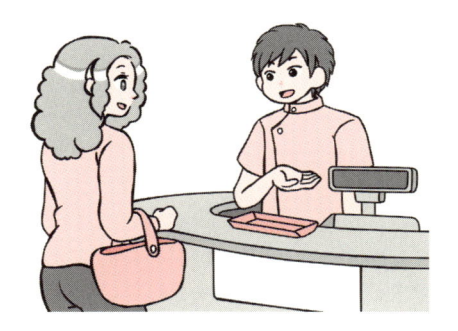

より丁寧 ↑ 丁寧さ

面会受付
Visitor's Counter

面	入院中の山田ジェーンさんに面会したいのですが.	I am here to visit Ms. Jane Yamada.
看	ご家族の方ですか？	Are you a family member?
面	いいえ．友人です．	No, just a friend.
看	ご家族以外の面会時間は午後1時からです．あと30分ほどお待ち頂けますか？(⇨ OP)	I am sorry, but visiting hours for people outside the family start from 1 PM. **Do you mind waiting 30 minutes**?
面	はい，わかりました．	Sure, I understand.
面	もう面会に行ってもいいですか？	May I go see her now?
看	はい，どうぞ．面会簿にお名前と時間をお書き下さい．ここから先はこのバッジをお付け下さい．お帰りの際にバッジは箱にお返し下さい．(⇨ OP)	Yes, go ahead. Please write your name and the time in the visitor's log. And please wear this visitor's badge during your visit. When you leave, **please put your badge in this box**.
面	はい，そうします．	OK, I will.
面	ありがとうございました（バッジを返す）．	Thank you. (returns badge)
看	ありがとうございます（⇨ Eric's Tip 8）．お友達はいかがでしたか？	Thank you. How was your friend?
面	思ったよりも元気で安心しました．	I'm happy because she is doing better than I expected.
看	それは良かったですね．お気をつけてお帰り下さい．	That's good news. Take care and have a safe trip home.

Optional Phrases

◘ あと30分ほどお待ち頂けますか？

I am sorry, but can you wait 30 minutes?
Would you mind waiting 30 minutes?
Do you mind waiting 30 minutes?
Can you wait 30 minutes?
You have to wait 30 minutes.（命令的）

より丁寧 ↑ 丁寧さ

◘ バッジ*は箱にお返し下さい．

Please bring your <u>badge</u> back and put it（複数の場合は them）in this box.
Please return your <u>badge</u> to this box.
Please put your <u>badge</u> in this box.

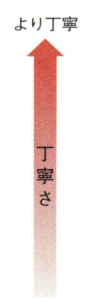

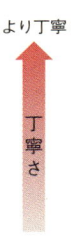

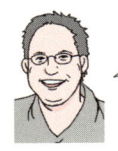

より丁寧 ↑ 丁寧さ

Eric's Tip 8　サンキューにはサンキューでも OK
"Thank you." と言われたら "You are welcome." と返事するものだと思われがちですが，状況によっては "Thank you." と答える方が自然です．

---

* 書類（forms），診察券（patient ID card），タオル（towel），ペン（pen）などの場合でも使えます．

2

診療科窓口
Department Reception Desk

受付・説明
Reception/Explanation

Track 14

看 おはようございます．初診の方ですか？(⇨ **OP**).	Good morning. **Is this your first time to come here**?
患 はい，初めて来ました．	Yes, it is.
看 **診察券とカルテをお出し下さい．**(⇨ **OP**).	**Please show me your patient ID card and chart(s).**
患 はい．	Here you are.
看 お預かりします．今日の初診担当は相沢医師です．問診表（付録B, p.152）にご記入下さい．記入が終わったらお出し下さい．	Thank you. Today your doctor will be Dr. Aizawa. Please fill out this questionnaire. When you're finished, please bring it to me.
患 はい．書きました．	Here you go.
看 順番でお呼びしますので，いすにかけてお待ち下さい．**申しわけありませんが**(⇨ **OP**)，今日は混雑しているので，初診の方には1時間ほどお待ち頂いています．	Please have a seat until we call your number. **I am afraid** we are pretty busy today. You will most likely wait for more than one hour.
患 1時間？ ここにいないといけませんか？	One hour? Must I stay here the whole time?

2. 診療科窓口

看 ほかの場所に行かれるときには受付に声をおかけ下さい．(⇨ **OP**)

If you are going to be somewhere else, please let us know when you leave.

患 わかりました．

Sure.

▶ Optional Vocabulary

カルテ　chart 常, patient file 常, clinical record 医

Optional Phrases

◘ 初診の方ですか？

Is this your first time to come to this department?
Is this your first time to come here?
Is this your first time here?

より丁寧
↑
丁寧さ

◘ 診察券とカルテをお出し下さい．

Please hand me your patient ID card and chart(s).
Please show me your patient ID card and chart(s).
Please give me your patient ID card and chart(s).

より丁寧
↑
丁寧さ

◘ 申しわけありませんが*…

I am sorry but as you can see, …
I am afraid, …
I am sorry, …

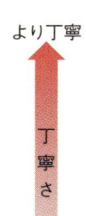

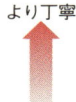

より丁寧
↑

---

* 患者さんに悪いことを知らせる場合に用いる丁寧な慣用句です．使った方がベターです．

◘ ほかの場所に行かれるときには受付に声をおかけ下さい.	If you are going to be somewhere else, please inform us when you leave.	より丁寧 ↑ 丁寧さ
	If you are going to be somewhere else, please let us know when you leave.	
	When you leave, be sure to tell us.	
	Before you leave, tell us.（失礼な表現）	

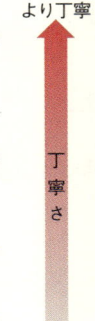

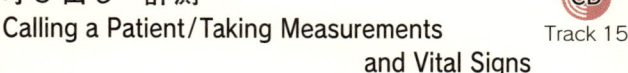

呼び出し・計測
Calling a Patient／Taking Measurements and Vital Signs

Track 15

看	モリスさん？ ナンシー・モリスさん.	Mrs. Morris?　Nancy Morris?
患	はい.	Yes?
看	お待たせしました(⇨ OP).中にお入り下さい.	**Thank you for waiting.** Please come inside.
患	はい.	OK.
看	まず身長と体重を計りますので，こちらにどうぞ.	First, we'll check your height and weight, so please come this way.
患	はい.	Alright.
看	身長を計ります．背筋を伸ばしてあごを引いて下さい．あなたの身長は172 cmです(⇨ OP).	Let's start with your height. Stand up straight and lower your chin. **You are 172 centimeters tall.**

患 ずっと変わりません.	Never changes.
看 体重計に乗って下さい. **体重は 74 kg です**(⇨ OP).	Next, please get on the scale. **You are 74 kilograms**.
患 嬉しいわ. 3 kg ほどやせました.	Great! I lost more than three kilograms.
看 つぎに血圧を計ります(⇨ OP). こちらにおかけ下さい. 上着を脱いで(⇨ OP), 右腕を出して下さい. 楽にしていて下さい. 124/80 mmHg です. 正常です(⇨ OP, Eric's Tip 9).	Now **we'll check your blood pressure**. Have a seat here and **please remove your shirt** and give me your right arm. Relax your arm. Your blood pressure is 124 over 80. **These are good numbers**.
患 よかったです.	That's good.
看 脈を計ります. 72 回/分です. 体温を測りますので, これを脇の下にしばらく挟んで下さい. 音がしたら取出して下さい.	Let's take your pulse...72. Let's take your temperature. Put the thermometer under your arm and keep it there. When it beeps, please take it out.
患 鳴りました.	I think it's beeping.
看 37.2 ℃です. 微熱がありますね.	37.2 degrees Celsius. You have a slight fever.

▶ Optional Vocabulary

微 熱　slight fever 常, mild fever 常

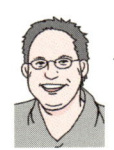

Eric's Tip 9　前向きな表現を使いましょう

血圧値が 124/80 mmHg のとき, 日本語では「正常です」と伝えるかもしれませんが, 英語で "This is normal." は平凡すぎる表現です. ネイティブスピーカーは "These are good numbers." のような前向きで肯定的な表現を好みます. 他のデータでも同じように表現してみましょう.

Optional Phrases

- お待たせしました. | Thank you so much for waiting. ← より丁寧
  Thank you for waiting. ↑ 丁寧さ
  Thanks for waiting.

- 身長は 172 cm です. | Your height is 172 centimeters.
  You are 172 centimeters tall.

- 体重は 74 kg です. | You weigh 74 kilograms.
  Your weight is 74 kilograms.
  You are 74 kilograms.
  You are 74 kilos.

- 血圧を計ります. | We'll check your blood pressure.
  We'll take your blood pressure.

- 上着を脱いで下さい. | Please remove your shirt.
  Please take off your shirt.

- 正常です. | You have a healthy blood pressure.
  These are good numbers.
  You are healthy.
  This is normal.

3

問 診
Brief Interview

問診・症状確認
Reviewing the Interview Sheet

Track 16

看 モリスさん，今日は発熱と咳と胸の痛みで受診されるのですね？	Mrs. Morris, I see you are here today because of a fever, cough, and chest pain. Is that right?
患 はい，そうです．	Yes, that is right.
看 3日前から症状があると問診表に書かれていますが，熱は何度でしたか？	You wrote here that your symptoms started three days ago. What was your temperature?
患 3日前から38度5分から39度の熱が続いています．その前から風邪気味だったのですが，熱は計っていません．	It was between 38.5°C and 39°C from three days ago. Before that I felt like I was coming down with a cold, but I didn't check my temperature.
看 家で何かお薬を飲みましたか？（⇨ **OP**）	**Did you take anything for it?**
患 市販の風邪薬を飲みました．	I took some OTC cold medicine.
看 効き目はありましたか？（⇨ **OP**）	**Did it help?**

患	飲むと熱は下がるのですが，咳は続いていました．	After I took it, my fever went down, but my cough continued.
看	今朝も飲んできましたか？	Did you take anything this morning?
患	はい，飲みました．たぶんそれで熱が少し下がったのだと思います．	Yes, I did. That may be why my temperature has gone down a little.
看	胸が痛むのですか？	How is your chest pain?
患	咳や深呼吸をすると痛くてつらいです．	It really hurts when I cough or breathe deeply.
看	あと少しで診察になります．それまで大丈夫ですか？	In a few minutes, the doctor will see you. Will you be OK until then?
患	はい．大丈夫です．(⇨ **Eric's Tip 10**)	Do I have a choice?

▶ Optional Vocabulary

風邪気味　coming down with a cold, catching a cold ／　市販薬　over-the-counter medicine, OTC medicine, medicine from a drugstore, non-prescription medicine

---

Optional Phrases

◘ 何かお薬を飲みましたか？	Did you take any medicine? Did you take any drugs? Did you take anything for it?	
◘ 効き目はありましたか？	Did your symptoms improve? Did it make you feel better? Did it help? Did it work?	より丁寧　↑　丁寧さ

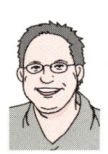

Eric's Tip 10　怒っているわけではない

"Do I have a choice?" とネイティブスピーカーが言っても，日本語の「仕方ないですね」くらいの意味で使うことが多く，怒っているわけではないので心配しないで大丈夫です．

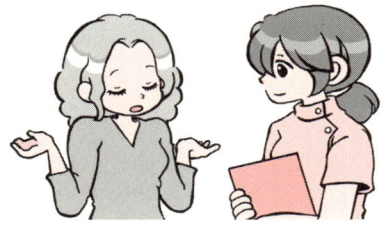

Do I have a choice?

4

診　察
Physical Examination

診察介助
Assisting Physician Examinations

Track 17

看	モリスさん．診察室5番にお入り下さい．	Mrs. Morris, please enter examination room number 5.
患	はい．	OK.
看	荷物は脱衣かごに入れて（⇨ OP），こちらのいすにお座り下さい．	**Please put your belongings into this basket**, and have a seat here.
患	どうも．	Thank you.
看	先生が胸の音を聞きますから，ブラウスの前ボタンを少し外して下さい（シャツの下を少しめくって下さい）．	For the doctor to check your breathing sounds, please undo a few buttons on your blouse (please lift your shirt up).
患	はい．	Alright.
看	楽にしていて下さい（⇨ OP）．つぎは背中から音を聞きますから，向きを変えて下さい．シャツの後ろを少しめくりますがよろしいですか？（⇨ OP）	**Please try to relax.** Next, she will listen from your back, so please turn around. **May I lift up your shirt**?
患	はい．	Yes, you may.

4. 診察

看	診察は終わりました．山下先生からの説明は理解できましたか？(⇨ **OP**)	Your examination is finished. **Were you able to understand Dr. Yamashita's explanation?**
患	はい．肺炎の疑いだそうです．検査の結果によっては，入院の必要があるそうです．	Yes, I was. She said I may have pneumonia and depending on my test results I may have to be hospitalized.
看	すぐに入院して頂いてもよろしいですか？	If need be, can we admit you to the hospital on short notice?
患	はい．必要であれば入院します．	Yes, you can.
看	では，これから血液検査とレントゲン検査を受けて頂きます．カルテと伝票を持って，まず向かい側の処置室へ行き，血液検査を受けて下さい．血液検査が済んだらレントゲン検査室に行って，終わったらここに戻ってきて下さい．	Next we are going to run some blood tests and take some X-rays. Here is your paperwork. Go across the hallway and you will have some blood taken. After your blood tests, you will go to the X-ray room. After your X-rays, please return here.
患	はい．わかりました．	I understand.

▶ Optional Vocabulary

入院する be hospitalized 常, check into the hospital 常, be admitted 医

Optional Phrases

◘ 荷物は脱衣かごに入れて下さい.

Please put your belongings into this basket.
Please put your things into this basket.
Put your stuff into this basket. (失礼な表現)

より丁寧 ↑ 丁寧さ

◘ 楽にしていて下さい.

Please make yourself comfortable.
Please try to relax.
Please don't worry.
Just relax.

◘ シャツの後ろを少しめくりますがよろしいですか?

Do you mind if I lift up your shirt?
May I lift up your shirt?
Is it OK to lift up your shirt?

より丁寧 ↑ 丁寧さ

◘ 山下先生からの説明は理解できましたか?

Were you able to understand Dr. Yamashita's explanation?
Were you able to follow Dr. Yamashita's explanation?
Could you follow Dr. Yamashita's explanation?
Did you understand what she said?
Did you get that?

より丁寧 ↑ 丁寧さ

5

処　置
Treatment & Procedure

創処置
Wound Treatment

Track 18

看 自転車で転んでけがをしたのですね(⇨ **OP**). それは痛かったことでしょう(⇨ **OP**).	**I heard you had a bicycle accident. I am sure that hurt.**
患 ええ，とても．段差で転んでしまいました．	Yes, it really does. I hit a big bump in the road and fell over.
看 けがをしたのは左膝だけですか？(⇨ **OP**) 頭や胸をぶつけてはいませんか？	**And only your left knee is injured? Did you hit your head or chest?**
患 大丈夫です．ヘルメットもかぶっていたので助かりました．	No, I didn't. Wearing my helmet really helped me.
看 傷口を洗浄しますから，処置室にお入り下さい．	In order to clean out your wound, we will move to the treatment room.
患 はい．	OK.
看 ズボンを脱いで，足をこの台の上に乗せて下さい．では傷口を洗浄します．	Please remove your pants and put your leg up on this table. Now I am going to clean out your wound.
患 この処置は痛いですか？	Will it hurt?

看 少しだけ痛いかもしれませんが，我慢して下さい（⇨ **OP**）．もう終わりました．あとはこの透明なテープを貼っておきます．	It's going to hurt a little. **Hang in there**. OK, we are done. Now I am going to put a clear bandage over the wound.
患 家に帰ってからシャワーを浴びてもよいのでしょうか？	May I take a shower when I get home? (⇨ **Eric's Tip 11**)
看 テープを貼ってありますから，シャワーで洗い流すならば大丈夫です．湯船には絶対につからないで下さい．	Because the bandage is waterproof, that will be no problem. However, please don't take a bath.
患 わかりました．ありがとうございました．	I see. Thank you.

▶ Optional Vocabulary

洗浄する　clean out 常, cleanse 常, irrigate 医

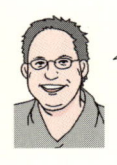

Eric's Tip 11　本当の男はお風呂が嫌い!?

日本人はたいていお風呂好きですから，思うようにお風呂に入れない入院生活は大変だと思います．欧米では「入浴するのは女性か子供」という強いイメージがあります．実際，欧米男性の多くは，湯船につからずに短時間のシャワーだけで済ませてしまいます．だからお風呂に入れなくても気にならないと思います．

Optional Phrases

- 自転車で転んでけがをしたのですね.

  I heard you injured yourself in a bicycle accident.
  I heard you had a bicycle accident.
  I see you had a bicycle accident.

- それは痛かったことでしょう.

  That must have been really painful.　より丁寧
  I am sure that was painful.
  I am sure that hurt.
  I bet that hurt.

  丁寧さ

- けがをしたのは左膝だけですか?

  And only your left knee needs treatment?
  And only your left knee is injured?
  And only your left knee is banged up?

- 我慢して下さい.

  Hang in there.
  Brace yourself.

注　射
Giving a Shot

Track 19

看 予防注射をしますから，左腕を出して下さい．	Now I am going to give you an immunization shot, please give me your left arm.
患 これでいいですか？	Like this?
看 はい十分です．少しチクッとしますよ．はい，もう終わりました(⇨ OP)．	Yes, thank you. This will sting a little. **OK, we're done.** (⇨ **Eric's Tip 12**)
患 ありがとうございました．	Thank you very much.
看 注射をしたところをもまないで下さい．出血するといけないので，絆創膏を貼っておきます．少ししたら剥がして下さい(⇨ OP)．	Please don't rub the area where I gave you the shot. Let's put a bandage on you to stop the bleeding. **After a little while, you should be able to remove it.**
患 わかりました．副作用の心配はありませんか？	I see. Do I have to worry about any side effects from the shot?
看 注射の跡が赤くなったり，腫れたり，痛んだりすることがありますが，数日で治ります．発熱や頭痛，全身の疲労感なども出ることがありますが，2,3日もすれば治ります．もし何かあれば，連絡して下さい(⇨ OP)．	There may be some reddening, swelling, or pain where I injected you; however this should go away after a few days. Some people experience fever, headaches, or fatigue, but these symptoms also go away after a few days. **If they persist, contact the hospital.**
患 今夜はお風呂に入ってもいいですか？	May I take a bath tonight?
看 はい．注射した部分をこすらないようにして下さい．	Sure. But don't scrub the area where I injected you.
患 助かりました．ありがとう．	I understand. Thank you.

▶ Optional Vocabulary

注 射　shot 常, injection 医／注射する　give a shot 常, give an injection 医／注射箇所(部位)　injection site 医／腫 れ　swelling, puffiness／疲労感　fatigue, tiredness, weariness, to be worn out

Optional Phrases

◘ はい，もう終わりました．	OK, we're done/finished here. OK, we're finished. OK, we're done. OK, I'm done. OK, we're done. Good job.（10歳以下の子供に対してだけ使う表現）	より丁寧 ↑ 丁寧さ
◘ 少ししたら剝がして下さい．	After a little while, you should be able to remove it. After a little while, you can take it off. In a little while, you can remove it. Wait a little before taking it off.	より丁寧 ↑ 丁寧さ
◘ もし何かあれば，連絡して下さい．	If they persist, feel free to contact the hospital. If they persist, contact the hospital. If they persist, give us a call. If they persist, just call.（失礼ではないが，くだけた表現）	より丁寧 ↑ 丁寧さ

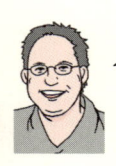

> **Eric's Tip 12　患者さんと何かするときは I よりも We**
> 医療現場では "I'm done." あるいは "I will put a bandage on you." と言うよりも，"We are done." "Let's put a bandage on you." と一人称は複数形で言った方がベターです．単数形 "I" では一方的に看護師が行う感じがします．その点，"We" と複数形にすれば，患者さんと看護師の両方の動作のニュアンスが出てきます．

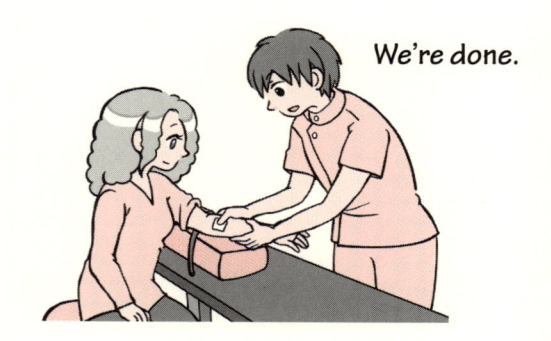

We're done.

6

診　察　後
After Examination

次回の外来診察予約・緊急時の連絡方法
Follow-up Exam/Emergency Contact

Track 20

看	クラークさん，次回の診察の予約をお取り下さい．ご都合はいかがですか？(⇨ **OP**)	Mrs. Clark, please make an appointment for your next visit. **What date and time is convenient for you**?
患	いつ来ればいいですか？	When would be a good time to come back?
看	来週の水曜日，25日の午後2時はいかがですか？	How about next Wednesday, the 25th, at 2 PM?
患	水曜日の午後は会議があるので，24日の火曜日に来てもいいですか？	I have a meeting to attend that Wednesday afternoon. How about the day before, Tuesday the 24th?
看	はい．でも24日の空いている時間は3時半になりますが，よろしいですか？	That should be OK, but our only available slot on the 24th is from 3:30. Will you be able to come in then?
患	大丈夫です．	That will be fine.
看	これが予約票です．次回，受付に診察券と一緒にお出し下さい．	Here is your appointment card. Please show this with your patient ID card at the front desk next time.

患	もしも次回までにまた具合が悪くなったら，どうしたらいいですか？	What should I do if I get sick again before my next visit?
看	**ご心配なく**（⇨ **OP**）．月曜日から金曜日の昼間でしたら，こちらにお電話下さい．夜間と休日は当直看護師が対応します．連絡先の電話番号は 03-7351-××××.*予約票にも書いてあります．	**Please be at ease.** During the daytime on weekdays, feel free to give us a call. At night and on weekends, nurses on call will be able to assist you. Our phone number is 03-7351-×× ××. It is also on your appointment card.
患	ありがとうございます．たぶん大丈夫だと思うのですが，それを聞いて安心しました．では来週の火曜日にまたお伺いします．	Thank you so much. I guess I will be all right until next week, and I am relieved to have your number. OK, I will be back next Tuesday.
看	**お大事にどうぞ**（⇨ **OP**）．	**Please take care**.

▶ **Optional Vocabulary**

具合が悪い　get sick, feel sick, feel bad, feel ill, don't feel good, be under the weather

---

* 電話番号の発音の仕方：0 はゼロのほかに ou（オー）とも発音します．"03-7351-××××" は zero three または ou three です．"045" のように，最初に来る 0 は zero で，それ以外は ou の発音が一般的です．"045" は zero four five と発音しますが，zero forty five とは決して言いません．"7351" は three seven five one とも発音しますが，2 桁ずつ発音することも多く，thirty seven fifty one と発音します．

Optional Phrases

◘ ご都合はいかがですか？
- What date and time is convenient for you? — より丁寧
- What day and time is convenient for you?
- When will be good for you?
- When can you make it?

◘ ご心配なく．
- Please be at ease. — より丁寧
- Please don't worry.
- Be at ease.
- Don't worry.

◘ お大事にどうぞ．
- I hope you get well soon. — より丁寧
- I hope you feel better soon． / Please take care.
- Get well soon.
- Have a nice day.
- Take care.

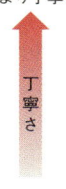

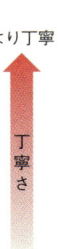

処方箋と薬局
Prescriptions and the Pharmacy

Track 21

看	クラークさんですか？ (⇒ OP)	Are you Mrs. Clark?
患	はい，そうです．	Yes, I am.
看	山田先生から説明があったと思いますが，抗生剤の処方箋が出ています．	As Dr. Yamada explained to you, she has prescribed you some antibiotics.
患	はい，伺っています．	Yes, that's what she told me.
看	お薬は院外の薬局で受け取って下さい．行きつけの薬局はありますか？	Please take this prescription to a pharmacy and they will fill it. Is there a pharmacy that you regularly go to?
患	行きつけではないのですが，家の近くに薬局はあります．	I do not go there often, but there is one near my house.
看	会計の近くにある院外処方箋コーナーから処方箋をファックスで送信しておけばすぐに受け取ることができますよ．	If you send this prescription to that pharmacy from the fax machine near the cashier's counter, your meds will be waiting for you. (⇒ Eric's Tip 13)
患	本当ですか．それは便利ですね．では，そうすることにします．	Is that so? That is really convenient. I will be sure to use your fax.

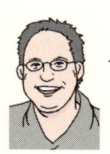

Eric's Tip 13　Meds は薬のこと

一般に使われている表現がいつも辞書に出ているとは限りません．たとえば，米国の医療従事者のほとんどが"meds"という表現を使います．これは"medicine"や"medication"の短縮形です．"meds"は複数形に見えますが，単数にも複数にも使います．単数形で"med"と言った場合は"medical"の略です．患者さんが米国人だったら，思い切って"meds"を使ってみましょう．

Optional Phrases

◩ クラークさんですか？

Excuse me, is your name Mrs. Mary Clark?

Excuse me, are you Mrs. Clark?

Are you Mrs. Clark?

Is your name Clark?（失礼な表現）

Clark?（とても失礼な表現）

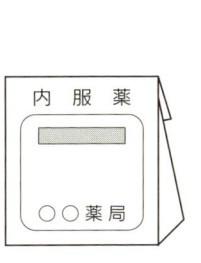

より丁寧 ← 丁寧さ

診断書の発行
Issuing a Medical Certificate

Track 22

患 保険会社に提出するので，診断書を頂けますか？
Can I get a copy of my medical certificate for my health insurance company?

看 決まった書式がありますか？
Is there a form that needs to be filled out?

患 はい，これです．
Yes, here it is.

看 この申込書にまずご記入下さい．記入できたら，お持ちの書類と一緒に1階の窓口にお出し下さい．
Here's an application form, please fill it in. After you are finished, please take it and your form to the 1st floor.

患 診断書の料金はいくらでしょうか？
How much will the medical certificate cost me?

看 ここに各種文書の料金表があります．所定の様式の診断書ですと，当院では5000円です．
Here's a chart with the prices for various forms. The medical certificate you need will cost you 5,000 yen.

患 あらま！ 意外と高いのですね？ 今日中に頂けるのでしょうか？
Wow! Isn't that a lot? Can I get it today?

看 いいえ．1, 2週間かかると思います．郵送をご希望であれば，その旨を受付に伝えて下さい．
I'm sorry, but I think it may take 1-2 weeks. If you prefer it mailed to you, just let the staff know when you order it.

患 わかりました．ありがとう．
Alright, thanks.

7 入院手続き
Hospitalization Procedure

入院案内
Hospitalization/Admissions Explanation
Track 23

看 モリスさん，8階病棟に入院して頂きます．今日はどなたかご一緒においでですか？(⇨ **OP**)

Mrs. Morris, you are going to be admitted to the 8th floor of our hospital. **Did someone accompany you today?**

患 いいえ，ひとりで来ました．これから夫に電話で入院を知らせますので，まもなく来てくれると思います．

No, I came by myself. I plan on calling my husband and letting him know that I am going to be in the hospital. I am sure he will be here soon after that.

看 ご主人のお勤め先はここから近いのですか？(⇨ **OP**)

Is your husband's place of work nearby?

患 家の隣に仕事場があります．

Actually, his workplace is near our home.

看 そうですか(⇨ **OP**)．では，病院のすぐ近くですね．今日は印鑑をお持ちですか？

Is that so? That is convenient. Did you bring your *hanko* with you?
(⇨ **Eric's Tip 14**)

患 はい，持っています．

Yes, I did. It's right here.

看 では，入院受付に少し寄って手続きをお手伝いします．それから病棟にご案内します．

First, we will stop by the admissions desk. I will help you do some paperwork. Then, I will show you to the ward.

▶ Optional Vocabulary

病棟　ward, floor, unit, patient care unit

Optional Phrases

◘ 今日はどなたかご一緒においでですか？	Did you come with a family member? Did someone accompany you today? Are you here with anyone?
◘ ご主人のお勤め先はここから近いのですか？	Does your husband work near here? Is your husband's place of work nearby? Is your husband's office nearby? Is your husband's company near here?
◘ そうですか．	Is that so? Is that the case? Is that right? Is that true?

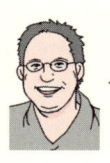

Eric's Tip 14　Hanko で通じます
日本に住んで正式に働いた経験のある人はきっと印鑑（"hanko"で通じます）を持っているはずです．日本の印鑑に代わるものが欧米では署名です．

個室料金
Private Room Fee

Track 24

看 入院は初めてですか？	Is this your first time to be hospitalized?
患 はい．日本では初めてなので，ちょっと心配です．	It's my first time in Japan, so I am a little worried.
看 ご心配ですよね (⇨ **OP**)．でも，スタッフみんなでお手伝いしますので，何でもご相談下さい．	**I know how you must feel.** However, the staff will try to help you and feel free to ask questions anytime.
患 ありがとうございます．あなた方がいてくれて，とても心強いです．	Thank you so much. You are a true professional.
看 病室は4人部屋が基本です．8階病棟には有料の2人部屋と個室がありますが，ご希望になりますか？	In general, the patient rooms are four to a room. However, on the 8th floor they have both rooms for two and private rooms for an extra fee. What's your preference?
患 4人部屋は無料ということですか？	Are the four-person rooms free?
看 いいえ，そういう意味ではなくて，4人部屋には保険が適応されます．2人部屋は1日2100円の自己負担が必要です．個室には3タイプありますが，空いているのは1日13,650円のBタイプです．	Oh, I am sorry, that's not what I meant. A four-person room will be covered by your insurance. A two-person room will cost an extra 2,100 yen per day out-of-pocket. As for the private rooms, we have three types. Currently, we have only one type — the B type — available at an extra 13,650 yen per day.

患	それでは，個室をお願いします．	If that's the case, I'll take the private room.
看	わかりました．個室を利用される場合は，申込書にご記入頂きます．ご面倒ですが，よろしくお願いします(⇨ **OP**)．	OK. To use a private room, please fill out this form. **I know it's a pain, but we appreciate your understanding.**
患	日本では，入院するためには，書類がたくさんありますね．	There sure a lot of forms that have to be filled out when getting hospitalized in Japan.

▶ Optional Vocabulary

4人部屋　four (patients) to a room, four-patient room, four-person room

---

Optional Phrases

❏ ご心配ですよね．	I can't imagine how stressful this must be for you. I know how worried you must be. I know how you must feel. I am sure you must be worried. I know how you feel.	より強い ↑ 共感の強さ
❏ ご面倒ですが…	I know it's a pain, but… I understand it's troublesome, but… I know I am asking a lot, but… I understand it's irritating, but…	

◪ …，よろしくお願いします．

..., but we appreciate your understanding.
..., but this will help us help you.
..., but we really need this done.
..., but it can't be helped.

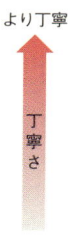

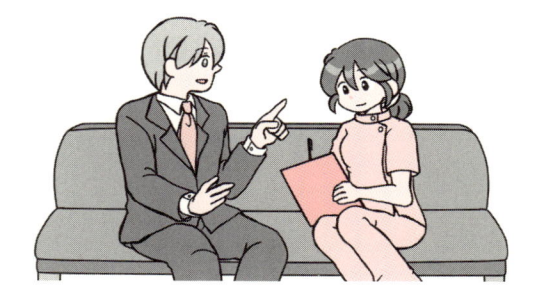

より丁寧

丁寧さ

入院時持ち物
Checklist of Items for Hospital Admission

Track 25

看	ここにご用意頂くもののリスト(付録C, p.156)があります.	Here's a list of everything you should prepare for your stay in the hospital.
患	わぁ,たくさんの荷物になりますね.洗面器まで持ってくるのですか?	Wow! That's a lot of stuff! I even have to bring a washbowl?
看	ええ,申しわけありません.	I am afraid that's right.
患	寝具も持参する必要がありますか?	Is it necessary for me to bring my own bedding?
看	いいえ,寝具は病院で用意します.入院料金に含まれております(⇨ **OP**).	No, we will supply you with bedding. **It is all included in your hospitalization fees**.
患	寝巻は?	What about pajamas?
看	ご自分でお持ちになられてもいいですし,1日100円でご用意もできます.ご希望であれば,申込書を提出して下さい.	You may bring your own pajamas, or we can provide them for you for 100 yen a day. If that is what you prefer, please submit a request form.
患	寝巻にも申込書がいるのですか?	Do I really need to fill out a form for pajamas?
看	そうなんです.盗難の恐れがありますので,貴重品や多額の現金はお持ちにならないようにして下さい.(⇨ Eric's Tip 15)	I am afraid so. Please don't bring a large amount of cash or valuables with you as there have been a number of thefts.
患	はい,気をつけます.	I see and I will follow your advice.

▶ Optional Vocabulary

寝 巻　pajamas, sleep wear, night gown(女性物)

7. 入院手続き　55

Optional Phrases

◘ …は入院料金に含まれております．

...is/are all included in your hospitalization fees.

...is/are covered by your hospitalization fees.

...is/are covered by your insurance.

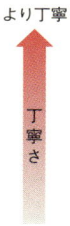

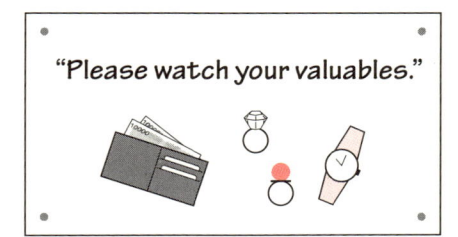

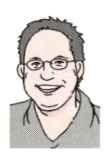

より丁寧 ↑
丁寧さ

"Please watch your valuables."

Eric's Tip 15　日本の安全神話の崩壊

滞在期間の短い欧米人だと，日本は安全だというイメージをもっているので，病院で盗難があるというのは驚くかもしれませんね．でも，大事なことなので，きちんと伝えておきましょう．

8

救 急 外 来
Emergency Room

救急患者への最初の確認
Initial Assessment of Emergency Patients Track 26

看	聞こえますか？ お名前を教えて下さい(⇨ **OP**).	Can you hear me? **Can you tell me your name**?
患	デービッド・グリーンです．	It's David Green.
看	デービッド・グリーンさんですね．目を開けて下さい(⇨ **OP**)．ここがどこかわかりますか？	OK, David Green. **Can you open your eyes**? Do you know where you are?
患	どこですか？ なぜ私はここにいるのですか？	Where am I? Why am I here?
看	ここは御江戸病院の救急外来です．駅前で突然倒れたので，救急車で運ばれてきたのです．先ほど，処置や検査をしました．	You are in the emergency room of the Oedo hospital. You fainted in front of the station, and an ambulance brought you here. We have already treated you and done some tests.
患	駅前で倒れたのですか？	I blacked out in front of the station?
看	ええ，そのようです(⇨ **OP**)．私の手を握ってみて下さい．	**Yes, that's what I am told.** Can you squeeze my hand?
患	これでいいですか？	How's this?
看	ええ，大丈夫です(⇨ **OP**)．	**Very good.**

患 妻に連絡してもらえますか？	Can you call my wife?	
看 はい．ご連絡先を教えて下さい．	Yes. Can you tell me her phone number?	

▶ Optional Vocabulary

突然倒れる   suddenly fall 常, black out 常, faint 常, pass out 常, experience syncope 医, lose consciousness 医

Optional Phrases

◘ お名前を教えて下さい．	Can you tell me your name? What's your name? Say your name. （緊急時のみ）	より丁寧　丁寧さ
◘ 目を開けて下さい．	Can you open your eyes? Can you look at me? Open your eyes. （緊急時のみ）	より丁寧　丁寧さ
◘ ええ，そのようです．	Yes, that's what I am told. Yes, that's what I heard. Yes, that's what they are saying. Yes, that's what they told me.	
◘ ええ，大丈夫です．	Excellent. Great job. Very good. That's good. That's OK.	より強い　ほめ方の強さ

家族への説明
Explanation to the Family

Track 27

看	デービッド・グリーンさんのご家族ですか？(⇨ OP)	**Are you a member of David Green's family?**
家	はい，そうです．お電話を頂いたので，急いで来ました．	Yes, I am. Thank you for calling me. I came as soon as I could.
看	さぞ驚かれたことでしょう．	I am sure this must be shocking to you.
家	ええ，びっくり．夫は大丈夫ですか？	Yes, I am so surprised. Is my husband OK?
看	はい．意識もはっきりされていますし，けがも全くありません．	Yes, he is. He is conscious and he has no injuries.
家	本当ですか．よかったです．いつ家に帰れますか？	Really? I am so happy to hear that. When can he come home?
看	一晩様子を見るために入院して頂きます．先ほど2階の病室に移りましたので，今からご案内します．	We are going to keep him overnight for observation. He has been taken to a room on the second floor; I will take you there now.
家	診察された医師とお話できますか？	Will I be able to talk to his doctor?
看	はい．でも，今は他の患者さんの診察中ですので，**診察が終わりしだい**(⇨ OP)，担当医がご説明します．	Yes, you will. But I am afraid his doctor is seeing to other patients at the moment. **When the doctor is finished**, she will explain things to you.
家	わかりました．	I see.

Optional Phrases

◘ ～さんのご家族ですか？

Are you a member of ～'s family?
Are you a relative of ～'s?
Are you related to ～?
Are you family?

◘ 診察が終わりしだい…

When the doctor is finished seeing to other patients...
When the doctor is finished seeing other patients...
When the doctor is finished with other patients...
When the doctor is finished ...
As soon as the doctor gets a chance...
When the doctor gets a chance...
As soon as the doctor has time...

より丁寧

丁寧さ

III

一般病棟

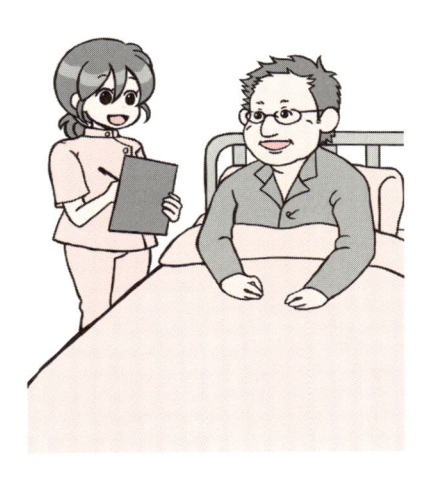

9 入　　院
Admission

自己紹介
Self-introduction

CD Track 28

看	(ノック後) こんにちは，入ってもよろしいですか？	Good afternoon, may I come in?
患	はい，どうぞ．	Sure.
看	失礼します．ナンシー・モリスさん．担当看護師の佐藤です (⇒ OP, Eric's Tip 16)．よろしくお願いします．	Sorry to bother you, Mrs. Nancy Morris. **My family name is Sato**, and I am going to be your nurse. It's a pleasure to meet you.
患	佐藤さんですね．こちらこそよろしく．	It's a pleasure to meet you, too, Sato-san.
看	副担当の看護師は宮沢です．今日は夜勤ですので，あとでご挨拶にお伺いする予定です．	Another nurse will also be caring for you*, and her name is Miyazawa. She's going to be working tonight and she will introduce herself to you later.
患	副担当は宮沢さん．わかりました．佐藤さんと宮沢さんが毎日担当して下さるのですか？	The name of another nurse caring for me is Miyazawa-san, I see. Will it only be the two of you looking after me every day?

---

* 日本語では"看護する"とあえて表現しませんが，英語では必要になります．

9. 入院

看 残念ながら，そうもいきません．昼間は私か宮沢看護師が担当させて頂きます．でも二人ともが夜勤の日には，ほかの看護師が来ます．私たちは**綿密に連絡を取合っています**（⇨ OP ）から，ご安心下さい．	I am afraid not. It will be either Miyazawa or me, but if we both work in the evening, another nurse will be looking after you in the daytime. **We have good lines of communication**, so please don't worry.
患 それを聞いて安心しました．	Well, I am relieved to hear that.

▶ Optional Vocabulary

看護する　care for, take care of, look after

Optional Phrases

○ 佐藤です．
　　My family name is Sato.
　　My last name is Sato.
　　Please call me Sato.
　　Just call me Sato.
　　I am Sato.

より丁寧 ↑ 丁寧さ

○ 私たちは綿密に連絡を取合っています．
　　We have good lines of communication.
　　We keep in touch on a regular basis.
　　We exchange information regularly.
　　We keep one another informed at all times.

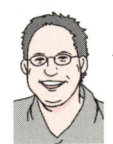

Eric's Tip 16　名字の伝え方

日本に長く住んでいる欧米人ならば別ですが，来日したばかりの人に "My name is Sato." と自己紹介すると，Sato をファーストネームと勘違いしてしまうかもしれません．ですから "My family name is Sato." と言いましょう．名字が Sato であることが確実に伝わります．

大部屋の案内
A Four-patient Room

Track 29

看	ここが307号室です．4人部屋です．	Here's room 307. It's a four-person room.
患	はい．	I see.
看	入って右側がグリーンさんのベッドです．	As you enter, the first bed on your right will be your bed, Mr. Green.
患	窓側ではないのですね．	I don't get to be next to the window?
看	明日，窓側のベッドが空く予定ですから，そうしたら移動しましょう．	Actually, from tomorrow a window-side bed will be available. Would you like to move to that bed tomorrow?
患	ええ，そうして下さい．	Yes, please.
看	お部屋の皆さんをご紹介しますね．前が山田さん，お隣が明日退院される川村さん，向こう側が森さんです．	I will now introduce your roommates to you. In front of you is Yamada-san, and next to the window is Kawamura-san, who is scheduled to be discharged tomorrow, and across from him is Mori-san.
患	(日本人)どうぞよろしく．	Do-zo yo-ro-shi-ku.
看	ベッドの間に仕切り用のカーテンがありますが，昼間はなるべく開けておいて下さい．	Between the beds is a curtain, however during the day please keep your curtain open.
患	わかりました．	OK.

病棟案内
Showing Around the Hospital Floor

看	ジョンソンさん,今から病棟をご案内しますが,よろしいですか?	Hello, Mrs. Johnson. If you don't mind, I will show you around this floor.
患	ええ,お願いします.	Yes, please.
看	両側の廊下の突当たりには非常口があります.ご確認下さい(⇨ **OP**).	At both ends of the hall you will find the emergency exits. **Can you see them**?
患	はい.	Yes, I can.
看	ここがナースステーションです.病棟を離れる際にはここの看護師に声をおかけ下さい.	And here's the nurses' station. If you are going to another floor in the hospital, please be sure to let someone here know.
患	はい,みなさん忙しそうですね.	Will do. Wow! Everyone looks so busy.
看	でも遠慮なさらずにいつでも声をかけて下さい.トイレと洗面所はここです.	Even so, please feel free to approach us anytime. And here's the bathroom with a sink for washing your hands and face.
患	トイレは和式ですか?	Are the toilets Japanese style?
看	いいえ,全部が洋式ですからご安心下さい.(⇨ **Shigemi's Tip 1**)	Nope, all of our toilets are western style. Please don't worry.
患	よかったです.	It's so nice!
看	ここがサンルームです.面会の方が一度にたくさん来られたときには,病室ではなくここでお話し下さい.	And here is a sunroom. If you have a number of visitors at the same time, we recommend you meet them here.
患	はい,わかりました.	OK, I see.
看	ここがお風呂場です.順番で	Here's where you can take a

20分ずつ使って頂いていますので，順番が来たらお使い下さい．	bath. The patients all take turns and get 20 minutes to bathe. Please go when it's your turn.
患 毎日使えますか？	Can I take a bath every day?
看 ええ．お風呂場を使えずに，ベッドで体を拭くだけの患者さんも多くいますから，毎日使って頂けると思います．でも時間は毎日いろいろだと思います．	Sure. Since some of the patients get bed baths, I think you should be able to take a bath every day. However, I think your bath time may differ from day to day.
患 毎日使えればそれで十分です．	Just as long as I can take a bath every day, I will be fine.

▶ Optional Vocabulary

ベッドで体を拭く（清拭）　bed bath（略して BB），sponge bath

Optional Phrases

❏ ご確認下さい．（方向を示しながら使う表現）	Are you able to see them from here? Can you see them? Make sure you know where they are. Make sure you know where it is.	より丁寧 ↑ 丁寧さ

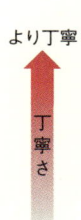

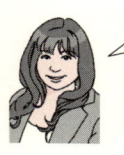

Shigemi's Tip 1　トイレは和式？ 洋式？

欧米人にとって，和式トイレは非常に使いにくいものです．洋式と和式の両方がある場合，どれが洋式トイレであるかを伝えましょう．大柄な患者さんの場合，日本の個室はかなり窮屈かもしれません．もし設備があれば，身障者用トイレを紹介しましょう．

10

オリエンテーション
Orientation

ベッド回りなど
Things Around the Bed

Track 31

看 ナースコールはここです．何かご用のあるときに押してお話し下さい．

Here is the nurse call button. If you need anything, please push it and then you can talk with us.

患 わかりました．着替えやタオルなどは，どこにしまえばいいですか？

I see. Where should I put my clothes and towels?

看 このロッカーと床頭台をお使い下さい．

Please use this locker and the cabinet next to your bed.

患 思ったよりも収納場所がありますね．シーツは毎日交換してくれるのですか？

There's quite a bit of space for my things. Will my bed sheets be changed every day?

看 いいえ．シーツは週に一度，毎週火曜日が交換日です．

I'm sorry, but they will be changed once a week on Tuesdays.

患 えっ，本当ですか？ 米国の病院では毎日換えると思います．

Really? In America I am pretty sure they are changed every day.

看 米国と同じようにサービスできなくて，申しわけありません（⇨ **Eric's Tip 17**）．

I am sorry, but we can't offer the same service as in America.

患	消灯時間はいつですか？	What time do I have to go to bed?
看	消灯は夜9時です．9時以降に灯りが必要であればこのスタンドをお使い下さい．	The lights will be turned off at 9 PM. If you need to use a light after 9 PM, please use this lightstand here.

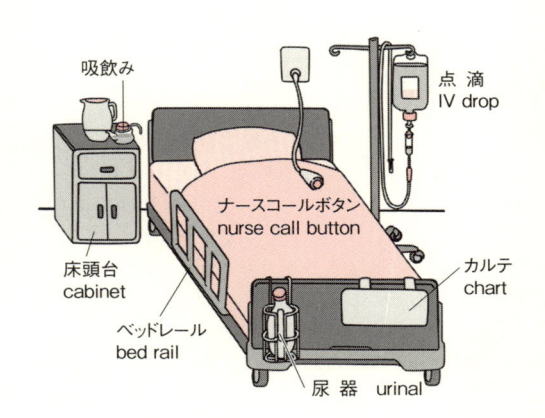

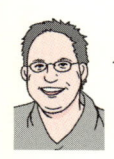

- 吸飲み
- 点滴 IV drop
- ナースコールボタン nurse call button
- 床頭台 cabinet
- カルテ chart
- ベッドレール bed rail
- 尿器 urinal

Eric's Tip 17 「ここは日本！」なんて言わないで

日本と自国とのさまざまな違いに患者さんは驚くことも多いはず．そんなときに，決して"This isn't America/the UK.（ここは米国/英国ではありませんから）"とは言わないようにしましょう．患者さんは疎外感を感じてしまいます．むしろ"I am sorry, but we can't offer the same service as in America/the UK."のように，共感的に受け止めましょう．

電　話
Telephone

Track 32

患	病院では携帯電話を使ってはいけないって本当ですか？	Is it true that I won't be able to use my mobile phone in the hospital?
看	ええ，院内ではお使いになれません．電話をおかけになるときは，階段脇のカード式公衆電話をお使い下さい．	I'm afraid so. Their use isn't permitted in the hospital (⇨ Eric's Tip 18). If you need to make a call, please purchase a phone card and use the pay phone near the stairwell.
患	カード式ですか？	What do you mean by "card"?
看	テレホンカード専用です．カードは２階の売店で販売しています．	The pay phones here use pre-paid cards. You can buy one at the shop on the 2nd floor.
患	あとで買いに行きます．もし家族が私に連絡を取りたいときはどうすればいいですか？	I will do that later. What if my family wants to contact me by phone?
看	ナースステーションに電話してもらって下さい．呼出しはできませんが，お電話があったことをすぐにお伝えするようにします．	They can call the nurses' station on this floor. We won't be able to let you talk to them, but we will give you a message from them.
患	それは助かります．ノートパソコンを持ってきているのですが，使ってもいいですか？	That's nice to know. I brought my laptop computer. Is it OK to use it while I am here?
看	パソコンは大丈夫です．こちらの電源をお使い下さい．でもお部屋のほかの方々に迷惑をかけないようにお願いします（⇨ OP）．	Sure. But please use this electric outlet only. And when using it in your room, **please be sure not to bother the other patients**.
患	はい，気をつけます．	I see. I will be careful.

▶ Optional Vocabulary

携帯電話　cell phone, cellular phone, mobile phone, smart phone

Optional Phrases

❏ ほかの方々に迷惑をかけないようにお願いします。

Please be sure not to bother the other patients.
Please don't be a nuisance to the other patients.
Please don't bother the other patients.
Don't bother the other patients.

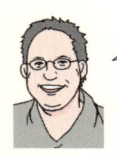

より丁寧 ↑
丁寧さ

Eric's Tip 18　複数形が一般的です

日本人には，単数形と複数形や，a や an と the の冠詞の使い分けを苦手に感じる人が多いようです．院内の規定やルールでは "no pets allowed（ペット持込み禁止）" "no children allowed（子供の入室禁止）" "no shoes allowed（土足厳禁）" のように，名詞部分は一般的に複数形を使います．冠詞に迷ったときのために，以下のルールが役立ちます．《a は one (of many) を意味し，the は it (only one 特に) を意味する．》

食　事
Meals

(CD) Track 33

看 食事には一般食と治療食がありますが，ジョーンズさんには糖尿病食が出ます．	We provide two kinds of meals: regular diet and special needs. Mr. Jones, I see that you will be on a special diet for diabetics.
患 ええ，上野医師がそう言っていました．1600 カロリーですって．きっとお腹が空くと思うので，家族にときどき何か差入れしてもらってもいいですか？	That's right. Dr. Ueno told me to expect this. He said it would be 1600 calories a day. I'm sure I'm gonna feel hungry all the time (⇨ **Eric's Tip 19**). Would it be OK if my family brings me a little something from home every once in a while?
看 いいえ，それはダメです．血糖値を下げるために，**食事制限を守りましょう**(⇨ **OP**).	I'm sorry, but that won't be allowed. In order to lower your blood glucose level, **we need you to stick to a strict diet**.
患 そうですね．頑張ります．そういえば，夕食時間はいつですか？	That's right. I'll do my best. By the way, when is dinner?
看 夕食は 6 時です．朝食が 7 時 30 分，昼食は 12 時です．*	Dinner is at 6 PM. Breakfast is at 7:30 and lunch will be at noon.
患 食事時間になったらどこに行けばいいですか？	When it's time to eat, where should I go?
看 食堂はないので，お部屋で食べて頂きます．食事は厨房から配膳車で運ばれてきます．配膳車が病棟に到着したらお	As we don't have a dining room, you'll be eating here in your room. The patients' food is brought on carts. When the

---

* おぼえておきたい表現 **2** (p.73)参照．

	知らせしますので，取りに来て下さい．	cart comes to this floor, there will be an announcement. At that time, you will have to come and get your tray.
患	セルフサービスなのですね．片付けはどうしますか？	So, it's a kind of self-service. How about cleaning up after eating?
看	お食事が済んだら，下膳車にお返し下さい．	After you have finished eating, please return your tray to the cart.
患	はい，わかりました．食事時間が楽しみです．	OK, I see. I look forward to meal time.

▶ Optional Vocabulary

食 事　meal, food 常, diet 医

Optional Phrases

○ 食事制限を守りましょう．　　We need you to stick to a strict diet.
　　　　　　　　　　　　　　　You need to follow a strict diet.
　　　　　　　　　　　　　　　We need you on a healthy diet.
　　　　　　　　　　　　　　　You must be on a prescribed diet.

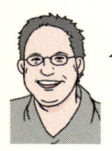

Eric's Tip 19　ワナ，ゴナ，ハフタ？

ワナ wanna (want to), ゴナ gonna (going to), ハフタ hafta (have to) は，口語英語で，ネイティブスピーカーがカジュアルな場面で使う，ごく自然な表現です．しかし，くれぐれも，公式の場では使わないようにしましょう．

おぼえておきたい表現
2 年号，日付，時刻の読み方

[年月日の記載]
- 記載順　米国: 月/日/年，英国: 日/月/年
  例: 1969 年 6 月 5 日
  米国　6/5/69 (six five sixty-nine)，英国　5/6/69

[年号の読み方]
1969 年　nineteen sixty-nine
2005 年　two thousand five

[日付の読み方]
1 日　first /　　2 日　second /　　3 日　third /
11 日　eleventh /25 日　twenty-fifth /30 日　thirtieth

[時刻の読み方]

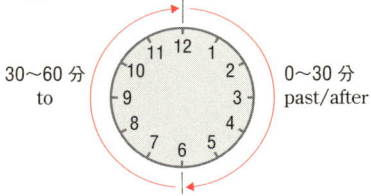

30〜60 分　　　　　　　　　　　0〜30 分
to　　　　　　　　　　　　　　past/after

30 分　past (after は使わない)

9:15	quarter past nine, quarter after nine
6:20	twenty past six, twenty after six
3:30	half past three (half after three とは言わない)
7:40	twenty to eight
11:55AM	five to noon
11:55PM	five to midnight

早朝検温
Early Morning Vital Signs Check

Track 34

看 チャンさん，おはようございます．	Good morning, Mr. Chan.
患 おはよう．	Good morning.
看 体温を計りましょう．これを脇に挟んで下さい．脈も取らせて下さい．	First, let's take your temp. Put this under your arm. And I'll also take your pulse.
患 はい，どうぞ．	Yes, please do.
看 脈拍数は72回/分，大丈夫です．昨夜はよく眠れましたか？	Your pulse is 72 beats per minute, which is good. Did you sleep well last night?
患 ええ，何かのアラーム音で2回ほど目が覚めましたけど，またすぐに寝ました．	Yeah, but some alarm went off twice last night and woke me up, but I went back to sleep soon after.
看 隣の輸液ポンプの調子が悪かったようです．申しわけありませんでした．お腹はまだ痛みますか？	The infusion pump over there is on the fritz. Sorry about that. Does your stomach still hurt?
患 ええ少しこの辺りが．体温計のビープが鳴りました．	Yeah, around here. The thermometer is beeping.
看 拝見します．体温は37.2℃．まだ微熱がありますね．吐き気はどうですか？	Let me have a look. Your temperature is 37.2. You still have a little fever. How is your nausea?
患 まったくありません．	Oh, I'm fine, thanks.
看 昨日，お通じはありましたか？	And did you have a bowel movement yesterday?
患 はい，2回ほど．少しゆるめでした．	Yes, twice. But they were a little loose.
看 そうですか．薬の影響がある	Is that so? It's probably a side

10. オリエンテーション

と思いますので,少し様子を見ましょう(⇨ **OP**).お小水には何回行かれましたか?	effect from your medicine. **I'll make a note of it.** How often did you urinate?
患 あまり覚えていませんが,7回くらいでしょうか.	I don't remember exactly, but around seven times.
看 お手洗いまで歩くのはつらくないですか?	Is it difficult to walk to the bathroom?
患 大丈夫です.	No, I'm OK.
看 朝食の後に内服薬をお持ちします.何かあったら,お知らせ下さい.	After breakfast, I'll bring you your meds. If you need anything, please let me know.
患 はい,ありがとう.	I will. Thank you.

▶ Optional Vocabulary

(機械の)調子が悪い　on the fritz 常, busted 男, broken 常, not working properly(丁寧な表現)

Optional Phrases

◘ 少し様子を見ましょう.	I'll make a note of it. We will see how things go. We will keep an eye on it/you. I will check again later.

午後の検温
Afternoon Vital Signs Check

Track 35

看	マーティンさん，3日前の夜に入院されたときにお会いした宮本です．今日の担当です．よろしくお願いします．	Hello Mrs. Martin. I'm Miyamoto, we met when you were admitted three days ago. Today, I will be your nurse. Nice to meet you, again.
患	こちらこそ，よろしく．しばらく夜勤をされていたのですね．	Likewise. You were working nights for a long time, weren't you?
看	ええ．今日から3日間は日勤です．ところで，咳は治まってきましたか？	Yes, I was. But now I have three day shifts in a row. By the way, how's your cough?
患	ありがとうございます．入院時に比べると随分と楽になりました．	Better. Thank you for asking. Since I was hospitalized, it has gotten much better.
看	朝食はどれくらいの量を召し上がりましたか？	How's your appetite at breakfast?
患	ほぼ全部食べました．	I've been almost finishing everything.
看	食欲も出てきましたね．良いことです．体温と血圧を計りましょう．脈も取らせて下さい．	Your appetite has returned! That's good news. Well, let's take your temp and check your blood pressure. I will also take your pulse.
患	はい，どうぞ．	Yes, please do.
看	血圧は150/96，脈拍数は66回/分，体温は36.7℃．血圧が少し高めですが，頭痛はしませんか？	Your blood pressure is 150/96, pulse is 66 beats per minute, and temperature is 36.7. Your BP is a little high. Do you have a headache?
患	いいえ，何とも．	No, not at all.

看 では,少し様子を見ましょう.もしも何か変わったことがあったら知らせて下さい.	OK, I'll make a note of it. However, if anything changes, please let me know.
患 はい,わかりました.	Yes, I will.
看 今日は午前中に胸のレントゲン写真を撮ることになっています.検査はもう済みましたか?	This morning you had a chest X-ray taken. Have you finished your other exams?
患 いいえ,なかなか呼出しがないので心配しています.	No, and I am a little worried as they haven't called for me.
看 そうですか.今日は検査を受ける人が多いのかもしれませんね.検査室に問合わせてみますので,もうしばらくお待ち下さい.	Is that right? There are probably a lot of people waiting for exams today. I'll go check with the people in the exam room and see what is going on. Please wait just a little longer.
患 はい,お願いします.	Yes, and thanks for checking.

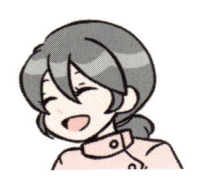

外出許可
Permission for Brief Leave

Track 36

| 患 | 入院が少し長引きそうなので，今日中に会社に行ってあれこれ調整してきたいのですが，いいですか？ | Since my stay here is going to be longer than I expected, I would like to visit my office to take care of some business. May I go today? |

| 看 | 外出には主治医の許可が必要です（⇨ **OP**）．回診のときに岡医師に相談してみましょう．それまでにこの"外出・外泊届"（付録D, p.158）にご記入下さい． | **In order to do so, you will need your doctor's permission.** When Dr. Oka comes by on rounds, please ask him. In the meanwhile, please fill out this form. |

| 患 | はい，そうします． | OK, I will. |

....

| 看 | スマイリーさん，正式に外出許可が出ました．これが許可証です．外出中はいつもお持ち下さい（⇨ **OP**）．何かあったらこの電話番号までご連絡下さい． | Mrs. Smiley, you have received permission to visit your office. Here is your permission card. **Please carry it with you at all times.** If anything happens, please call this number. |

| 患 | はい，わかりました． | OK, I see. |

| 看 | 外出先からお戻りになられたら，ナースステーションに声をかけて下さい． | Upon your return, please stop by the nurses' station and let us know. |

| 患 | はい．では行ってきます． | Will do. See you in a few hours. |

| 看 | お気をつけて．会社であまり無理をしないで下さいね． | Please be careful and don't work too hard. |

▶ **Optional Vocabulary**

許可 permission, consent, authorization, OK

10. オリエンテーション

Optional Phrases

◘ ～には主治医の許可が必要です.	In order to ～, you will need your doctor's permission.	より丁寧 ↑
	In order to ～, you should get your doctor's permisson.	丁寧さ
	In order to ～, you must get permission from your doctor.	
◘ いつもお持ち下さい.	You must have it on your person at all times.	より厳しい ↑
	Be sure to have it with you at all times.	厳しさ
	Please carry it with you at all times.	
	Please have it on you at all times.	

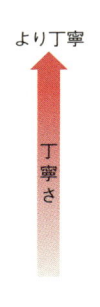

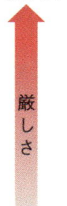

11 看護暦聴取
Nurse Interview

面接の導入
Starting the Interview

Track 37

看	ブッシュさん，こんにちは．担当看護師の佐藤です．よろしくお願いします．	Good afternoon Mrs. Bush. I am your nurse, Sato. Pleased to meet you.
患	こちらこそ，よろしく．	Likewise.
看	ブッシュさんの健康状態や健康管理についてお話をお聞きしたいのですが，今からよろしいですか？*	First, may I ask you some questions about your health and how well you take care of yourself?
患	はい，どうぞ．	Yes, go ahead.
看	今，ご気分はいかがですか？（⇒ OP）	Currently, **how are you feeling**?
患	酸素吸入を始めて頂いたので，少し楽になりました．	I feel much better after getting some oxygen.
看	室温はどうですか？　寒くないですか？	How is the temperature of your room?　Is it too cold?
患	そうですね，もう少し暖かくして頂けますか？	Actually, it is.　Could we make it a little warmer in here?

---

* 機能的健康パターンに基づくアセスメント項目は下記の書籍をご参照下さい．
Marjory Gordon, "Assess Notes", F. A. Davis (2008)；（日本語版）マージョリー・ゴードン 著，上鶴重美 訳，"アセスメント覚書"，医学書院 (2009)．

看	はい，わかりました．これから 30 分間ほどお話をお聞きするのですが，その前にお手洗いに行っておかれますか？	Sure. I have to interview you for about 30 minutes. Before that, would you like to use the ladies room?
患	ええ，そうします．	Yes, I will.
	………	………
患	お待たせしました．	Thank you for waiting.
看	では始めさせて頂きます．	Shall we start?

Optional Phrases

◘ ご気分はいかがですか？　　How are you feeling？ ← より丁寧
　　　　　　　　　　　　　　How are you doing？
　　　　　　　　　　　　　　How are you？

面接の終了
Finishing the Interview

Track 38

看	そのほかに何か話しておきたいことはありませんか？(⇨ OP)	**Is there anything else you wish to talk about**?
患	いいえ，今のところは思い浮かびません．	Nope, I've told you everything.
看	今一番つらいのは，痰のからむ咳だということがよくわかりました．田部井先生から1日4回のネブライザーの指示が出ています．その後にはしっかりと痰を出しましょう．痰を出しやすくするために，たくさん水分を取るようにしましょう．	I can see your phlegmy cough is bothering you the most. Dr. Tabei has you on a nebulizer four times a day. After that, be sure to cough up your phlegm. To help loosen your phlegm, be sure to drink a lot of fluids.

患	はい，わかりました．ではお茶を頂けますか？	I understand. By the way, can I get a cup of tea?
看	わかりました．部屋も乾燥しているようですから，加湿器を使いましょう．	Sure. Since your room is so dry, let's set up a humidifier.
患	ええ，お願いします．	Oh, thank you so much.
看	足が冷たいと言っておられたので，湯たんぽをお持ちします．	I remember you saying your feet were cold, would you like me to bring you a hot water bottle?
患	それは嬉しいです．	Oh, yes. That would be fantastic.
看	では，お茶と加湿器と湯たんぽを準備してきます．すぐに戻りますが，何かあれば，ナースコールをお使い下さい．	Alright, I am going to get some tea, a humidifier, and a hot water bottle. I will be back in a little bit. If you need something, please feel free to use the nurse call button.
患	わかりました．	I see.

▶ Optional Vocabulary

痰　phlegm [常], sputum [医]

Optional Phrases

◘ そのほかに何か話しておきたいことはありませんか？

Is there anything else you would like to share?

Is there anything else you wish to talk about?

Is there something else you wish to say?

Anything else?

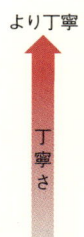

より丁寧 ↑ 丁寧さ

12

検 査 説 明
Explaining Exams

胃カメラ検査の説明
Explaining a Gastroscopy

Track 39

看	デカプリオさん、こんばんは．明日の検査について説明させて下さい．	Good evening, Mr. DiCaprio. I'm here to talk to you about tomorrow's exam.
患	明日は何の検査ですか？	What exam are you talking about?
看	10時から胃カメラ検査があります．以前にもこの検査を受けたことはありますか？(⇨ OP)	You will have a gastroscopy at 10 AM. **Have you had this exam before?**
患	ええ，5年ほど前に．苦しかったことを覚えています．	Yeah, I had one about five years ago. I remember it was really unpleasant!
看	それは大変でしたね．今回は楽に済むといいですね．(⇨ OP, Eric's Tip 20)	I'm sorry to hear that. **I hope it will be easier this time.**
患	本当にそう願います．	I sincerely hope so!
看	準備として，夜9時以降は何も食べないで下さい．明日の朝食も取れません．水は検査の2時間前まで飲んでも大丈夫です．水分補給は十分にし	To prepare, after 9 PM tonight, please don't eat anything. Further, you won't be having breakfast tomorrow morning. You may drink water until two

て下さい(⇨ **OP**).	hours before the exam. **Please be sure to get lots of fluids.**
患 朝の薬は飲まなくていいのですか？	So I won't be taking my meds tomorrow morning?
看 血圧のお薬だけは内服して頂きます．早朝に担当者がお持ちします．	You will only take your blood pressure pills. Your morning nurse will bring them to you.
患 わかりました．検査後しばらくの間は食べてはいけないのですよね？	I see. After my exam, I won't be eating anything for a while?
看 はい．検査後1時間程度は喉の麻酔が残っています．1時間くらいして，水を飲んでむせなければ，食べても大丈夫です．	That's right. You'll still be feeling the effects of the anesthetic. After about an hour, if you don't choke on water, we will let you eat something.
患 了解．	Gotcha[*].

▶ Optional Vocabulary

準備として　to prepare, to get ready, to get prepared

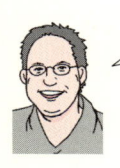

> **Eric's Tip 20**　"Pray"は慎重に使いましょう
> 宗教を大切にしている患者さんには"pray"を使って"I pray it will be easier this time."と言ってもいいのですが，そうでない患者さんには"hope"を使って"I hope it will be easier this time."と言いましょう．

---

[*] "Gotcha."は男性の使う表現で，女性ならば "I understand." "I see." "Got it."のように言います．

Optional Phrases

○ 以前にもこの検査を受けたことはありますか？
Have you had this exam before?
Have you ever had this exam before?
Have you ever experienced this exam before?
Have you ever undergone this exam before?

○ 今回は楽に済むといいですね．
I expect it will be easier this time.
I hope it will be easier this time.
I think it will be easier this time.
I pray it will be easier this time.

○ 水分補給は十分にして下さい．
Please be sure to get lots of fluids.
Please be sure to drink lots of fluids.
Please be sure to drink a lot of water.
Please be sure to take in plenty of liquids.

心臓カテーテル検査の説明
Explaining a Heart Cath Exam

Track 40

看 ローディングさん，先ほど原医師から明日の心臓カテーテル検査について説明があったと思いますが，理解できましたか？

Hello Mr. Rawding, I think Dr. Hara explained your upcoming heart cath exam, were you able to understand everything?

患 はい，大体．足の付け根の動脈から心臓まで管を入れて，血管が狭くなっている場所を調べると聞きました．

Yes, I understood most of what he said. I heard him say that the catheter would be inserted through the femoral artery in my groin to see which vessel is narrowing.

看 よく理解されていますね．検査について何かご心配なことはありませんか？

You understood really well! Do you have any worries about the exam?

患 心臓まで動脈から長いカテーテルを入れるなんて少し怖いです．それよりも，治療方針が早く決まった方がいいです．（早く決めた方がいいです．⇨ Eric's Tip 21）

I am a little afraid about a long catheter going from my groin to my heart. But, I will be better off deciding a course of treatment as soon as possible.

看 そうですね．検査は9時30分からの予定です．朝から何も食べられません．9時ごろに車いすで心カテ室までお連れします．

Yes, that's true. Your exam is scheduled for 9:30 AM. After waking up, please don't eat anything. At 9:00 you will be taken to the heart cath room in a wheelchair.

患 はい，わかりました．

I see.

看 検査は1時間ほどで終わりますが，検査後6時間は止血のためにベッド上で安静が必要です．その間はトイレに行け

The exam will take about an hour. And then you will lie flat on your bed for 6 hours to prevent bleeding. During that

ないので，尿器を使って頂きます．使ったことはありますか？	time, you won't be able to get up and go to the bathroom. So please use the urinal. Have you used one before?
患 いいえ，一度も．ずっと元気でしたから．	Nope, never. I've always been healthy up until now.
看 そうですか．寝たままの排尿はなかなか難しいので，一度，練習しておけば安心です．今度トイレに行きたくなったら，知らせて下さい．	Is that so? It's not easy to pee while lying flat, I recommend you try it once to see what it is like. Next time when you want to go to the bathroom, please call me.
患 今から行こうと思っているのですが．	Actually, I need to go now.
看 では，すぐに準備してきます．	OK, just a minute while I get everything ready.

▶ Optional Vocabulary

心臓カテーテル　heart cath 常, cardiac catheterization 医 ／ そけい部　groin 男, upper thigh ／ 尿器（しびん）　urine bottle 常, urinal 医

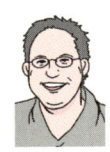

Eric's Tip 21　治療方針は誰が決めるのか？

欧米では医師が提示する複数の治療の選択肢から，最終的に決断するのは患者か家族なので，"But, I will be better off deciding a course of treatment as soon as possible. （治療方針を早く決めた方がいいです）" と言うのが一般的です．日本では治療方針を決めるのは医師なので，患者さんが「治療方針を決める」と言うことはほとんどないかもしれません．

13

治療・処置
Treatment & Procedure

点滴の差替え
Changing an IV Site

CD Track 41

看	リーさん，どうなさいましたか？	Mr. Lee, how can I help?
患	左腕の点滴の入っているところが何だかとても痛みます．	The area around the IV in my left arm is really sore.
看	どれどれ．あらほんと，赤くなっていますね．**炎症が起きてしまったのだと思います**（⇨ **OP**）．点滴を差替えましょう．	Let me have a look. You are right, it's pretty red. **There is some inflammation**. Let's change the IV site.
患	えっ，感染ですか？	Umm...is it infected?
看	感染のこともありますが，それは予防するように気をつけています．薬液の濃度や，pHや，血管に入れているカテーテルの刺激と，いろんな原因で炎症は起こると言われています．	Actually, we have been fighting the infection, so that's not it. Your inflammation may be due to the concentration of the drip, it's pH, or due to the catheter.
患	へえ，そうなんですか．	Is that so?
看	この点滴は抜きますね．…はい，抜きました．ここをしばらく押さえていて下さい．	I am going to remove your IV, OK? ...It's out. Please press here with your hand.

13. 治療・処置

患 はい．まだ点滴を続けなくてはダメですか？ — OK. Must I still have the IV?

看 十分な水分が摂れるまで，もうしばらく続けましょう．今から準備をしてきます．点滴のない間に，**着替えをされますか**？(⇨ **OP**) — I am afraid we have to continue the IV until you get well hydrated. While I go get a new IV kit, **why don't you change your clothes**?

患 ええ，そうします． — That's a great idea.

Optional Phrases

◘ 炎症が起きてしまったのだと思います．
- There is some inflammation.
- I see there is some inflammation.
- I see there is some reddening of the skin.

◘ …着替えをされますか？
- ...would you like to change your clothes? （より丁寧）
- ...why don't you change your clothes?
- ...do you wanna change your clothes?
- ...do you wanna change?

（丁寧さ）

▶ Additionary Vocabulary

注射 shot 常 ／ 輸液 transfusion 医 ／ 輸血 blood transfusion 医 ／ 完全静脈栄養（中心静脈栄養） total parenteral nutrition (TPN) ／ 中心静脈栄養 intravenous hyperalimentation (IVH) ／ 末梢静脈栄養 peripheral parenteral nutrition (PPN) ／ 経腸栄養 enteral nutrition ／ 筋肉注射（筋注） intramuscular injection (IM) ／ 点滴 intravenous injection (IV) 医，IV 常 ／ 皮下注射 subcutaneous injection (SC)

14

服 薬 指 導
Medication Instructions

服薬指導[*]
Medication Instructions

Track 42

看 ワンさん，今日から血圧を下げるお薬が変わります（⇨ OP）．以前の薬だと頭痛がしたそうですね．	Mrs. Wong, **from today we are going to change your blood pressure meds**. I heard your previous medicine was giving you a headache.
患 ええ，薬のせいかどうかわからないのですが，昨日渡辺先生にそうお伝えしました．	Well, I am not sure if my meds were causing my headaches. But I said yesterday to Dr. Watanabe that I was having headaches.
看 今はどうですか？	How are you today?
患 今は全く大丈夫です．	I am fine today.
看 それは良かったです．飲み方は以前の薬と同じです．1日1回1錠，朝食後に白湯かお水でお飲み下さい．	I am glad to hear that. You will be taking your new meds the same as your old meds. You will take one pill, once a day, after breakfast. Be sure to take it with water.

---

[*] 服薬指導の詳細は，下記の書籍をご参照下さい．
原 博，Eric Skier，渡辺朋子，"薬学生・薬剤師のための英会話ハンドブック"，東京化学同人(2009)．

患 以前の薬では，グレープフルーツを食べたりグレープフルーツジュースを飲んだりしてはいけないと言われましたが，今度の薬もそうですか？	I was told that I couldn't have grapefruit or drink grapefruit juice with my other medicine. How about this one?
看 今回の薬は作用が違うので大丈夫です．どんな薬にも副作用があるのですが，この薬のおもな副作用として，立ちくらみ，めまい，咳が知られているようです．何か変わったことがありましたら，教えて下さい．	This medicine works differently, so having grapefruit is OK. All medicines have side effects; this medicine's common side effects are to feel faint, dizziness, and a cough. If you experience any of these, please let us know.
患 わかりました．必ずお知らせします．	I see and I will be sure to let someone know.

▶ Optional Vocabulary

副作用　adverse effect(s)，adverse reaction(s)，side effect(s)，side-effect(s)*

Optional Phrases

❏ …今日から血圧を下げるお薬が変わります．	…from today we are going to change your blood pressure meds.	より丁寧 ↑ 丁寧さ
	…from today you will be on a new medication.	
	…from today we will put you on a new blood pressure drug.	

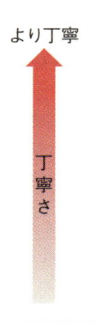

---

* ネイティブスピーカーは，ハイフンのある side-effect(s) もハイフンのない side effect(s) も両方使います．

15 栄 養 指 導
Nutritional Guidance

栄 養 指 導
Nutritional Guidance

CD Track 43

看	ソーヤーさん，今から少し食事についてお話しさせて頂いてもよろしいですか？	Mrs. Sawyer, I am here today to talk to you about your diet. Is that OK?
患	はい，どうぞ．	Yes, go ahead.
看	ところで，ソーヤーさんは，**腎臓の働きをご存知ですか？** (⇨ **OP**)	By the way, **do you know what your kidneys do**?
患	尿を作っているところ．余分な水分を出してくれているのだと思います．	Don't they make urine?[*1] They help the body get rid of excess water, I think.
看	ええ，そうですね．でも腎臓は水分だけではなくて，タンパク質が体の中で利用された後の老廃物，つまり有害物質も血液から沪過して体の外に	Yes, that's right. However, the kidneys not only do that, but also help remove poisonous waste products from your blood and protein use.[*2]

---

*1 "Don't they make urine?" と疑問形で表現していますが，質問ではありません．

*2 to の付かない不定詞を原形不定詞と言います．let, make, have などの使役動詞の目的格補語として用いられ，"使役動詞"＋"A: 人を表す目的語"＋"B: 原形不定詞"の形で，"A に B させる"の意味です．help は使役動詞ではありませんが，この構文に合わせて用います．[例]"I will help you ＋原形動詞"（口語では to を付けない．）

15. 栄養指導

出してくれているのです．	
患 タンパク質とも関係があるのですか．	So the kidneys and protein are related?
看 ええ．ほかにも，電解質の調節，造血ホルモンの分泌，血圧の調節，骨を作るのに必要なビタミンDの活性化といった働きもしてくれています．	Yes, they are. Your kidneys also help balance your electrolytes, produce your blood-making hormones, regulate your blood pressure, and are necessary to activate vitamin D to make your bones.
患 生きる上で欠かせない臓器なのに，私の腎臓は，あまり働かなくなってしまったのですね．	They sound like an invaluable organ, but mine aren't working so well, are they?
看 ええ，そうなのです．腎不全の患者さんの場合，今までのように好きなものを好きなだけ飲んで食べていたら，体に毒素がたまってしまいます．	I am afraid they aren't. In patients with kidney failure, if they eat and drink anything they like, hazardous products will accumulate in the body.
患 それは大変です．	That sounds like a bad thing.
看 ええ，だから，腎臓に負担をかけないような食事療法はとても大切です．ソーヤーさんの場合，特にタンパク質と塩分に気をつける必要があります(⇨ **OP**)．	Yes, it is. That's why it is important we put you on a special diet for your kidneys. In your case, **we have to pay special attention to your protein and salt intake**.
患 食べることがとても大好きなので，食事療法は辛いです．でも，自分の体のためですものね．頑張ってみます．	I really like food, so this diet is going to be hard. But, it is for my own good. I will do my best.

Optional Phrases

◘ …腎臓の働きをご存知ですか?
- …do you know what your kidneys do?
- …do you know why your kidneys are important?
- …do you know why you have kidneys?

◘ …特にタンパク質と塩分に気をつける必要があります.
- …we have to pay special attention to your protein and salt intake.
- …we have to control your protein and salt intake.
- …we have to watch your protein and salt intake.
- …we have to be careful about your protein and salt intake.

16

離床・リハビリテーション
Getting out of Bed & Rehabilitation

体位変換
Positioning

Track 44

看	ウエインさん，痛みはどうですか？	Hello Mr. Wayne, how's your pain?
患	痛くはないのですが，とても眠いです．	I don't feel any pain, but I am very sleepy.
看	薬が効いているためだと思います．でも同じ姿勢で長い時間寝ていると床ずれができてしまう危険があります．2時間ごとに体の向きを変えましょう．	I am pretty sure that is due to your meds. However, if you sleep in the same position for a long time, there is a risk of getting bed sores. It would be best for you to change your position once every two hours.
患	ええ，でも自分では動けそうもありません．	I understand, but I don't think I will be able to move on my own.
看	お手伝いしますから大丈夫です．ずっと仰向けでしたから，横向きになりましょう．まず少し腕の位置を変えます．	With a little help I think you'll be fine. You've been lying on your back for quite some time. Why don't we get you on your side? First, let's move your arm a little this way.
患	はい．	Yep.

看 次は足の位置を変えます。痛くはないですか？	Next, let's move your legs. Does that hurt?
患 大丈夫です。	I'm OK.
看 では最後に，体全体をこちらに向けましょう。体を楽にしていて下さい。1・2の3で（⇨ OP）向きを変えましょう。1・2の3，はい，できました。いかがですか？	And lastly, let's turn your entire body this way. Please relax and **when I say "three," we will** turn you to your left. One, two, three, and we're done. How's that?
患 ええ，腰が楽になりました。	That's nice. My back feels much better.
看 しばらくしたら，また来ます。次は反対側に向きを変えましょう。また少しお休み下さい。	After a while, I'll be back. Then we'll turn you facing the opposite direction. Please rest until then.
患 はい。ありがとう。	I will. Thank you so much.

▶ Optional Vocabulary

床ずれ，褥創　bedsore 常, pressure sore 常, pressure ulcer 常, decubitus ulcer 医

Optional Phrases

○ 1・2の3で…．　　　I will count one, two, three, and on three we will….
（詳しい説明が必要な人に対して使ってみましょう．）

…when I say "three," we will….
…on three, we will….

おぼえておきたい表現
3 体の向き・位置・姿勢を変える

左/右向きになって下さい.	Please turn to your left/right.
仰向け/うつ伏せになって下さい.	Please turn facing up/down.
こちらを向いて下さい.	Please face me.
向こう側を向いて下さい.	Please face the other way.
頭を右/左に向けて下さい.	Please turn your head to the right/left.
座って下さい.	Please sit up.
上の方に上がって下さい.	Please scoot up.
下の方に下がって下さい.	Please scoot down.
立ち上がって下さい.	Please stand up.
椅子の前/後の方に来て下さい.	Please scoot your chair up/back.
膝を曲げて下さい.	Please bend your knee(s).
足を伸ばして下さい.	Please extend your leg(s).
腕を曲げて下さい.	Please bend your arm(s).
腕を伸ばして下さい.	Please extend your arm(s).
腕をこんなふうに曲げて下さい.	Please bend your arm(s) like this.

車いす移動
Transferring to a Wheelchair

Track 45

看	ハワードさん，今日からリハビリが始まります．車いすに乗ってリハビリ室に行きましょう．	Hello Mrs. Howard, today we'll start your rehabilitation process. Let's get you in this wheelchair and go to the rehabilitation room. (⇨ **Eric's Tip 22**)
患	あちこち痛いので，あまり動きたくないのですけど．	I hurt all over and really don't want to move.
看	**痛みますよね**(⇨ **OP**)．でも，寝てばかりいると筋肉が弱ってしまいます．少しずつでも動かしましょう．	**I understand you're in pain**, but if you just sleep all the time, your muscles will weaken. Let's move you little by little.
患	ええ，そうですね．	Yes, I see what you're saying.
看	じゃあまず，体を起こしてみましょう．ベッドの頭の方を上げてみましょう．めまいはしませんか？	OK...first, let's get you up in bed. Let's start by adjusting the angle of the bed. Are you feeling dizzy at all?
患	いいえ．	Nope.
看	では次に，体の向きを変えて，ベッドの端に座ってみましょう．足を床につけて下さい．気分はどうですか？	Next, let's turn you around and get you on the edge of the bed. Please put your feet on the floor. How do you feel?
患	大丈夫です．	I'm OK.
看	では，横にある車いすに乗り移りましょう．私につかまって，首の後ろで手を組んで下さい．いいですか？	Now let's get you into this wheelchair. You are going to put your arms around my neck, and lock your hands together. Do you understand?
患	はい．	Yes.

看 ハワードさんの腰を支えますから掛け声で静かに立ち上がって下さい．立ち上がったら，体の向きを変えて，ゆっくりと車いすに座りましょう．わかりましたか？	Then I will support your hips and you should try to stand up on my count. After you are up, turn and we will lower you slowly into the chair. Do you understand?
患 はい．	Yep.
看 1・2の3で立ち上がりましょう．いいですか？	I will count one, two, three, and on three we will stand you up. Ready?
患 ええ．	Sure.
看 1・2の3(動く)．	One, two, three.

▶ Optional Vocabulary

筋肉が弱る　muscle loss 常，muscle atrophy 医

Optional Phrases

◯ 痛みますよね．	I understand you're in pain. I am sure you're in pain. I am sure you're hurting all over. I know it hurts, but…. I am sure it hurts, but….

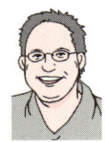

Eric's Tip 22　リハビリには愛のムチ

"Let's get you in …."は自然な英語ですが，あまり丁寧な表現ではありません．しかし，リハビリに関しては，患者さんの自主性が求められるので，Pleaseを使う必要はありません．欧米のリハビリでは"Tough love(愛のムチ)"が基本です．

17 患者家族へ
Talking to the Family of a Patient

家族の付添いについて
Visitor(s) Stay Overnight

Track 46

家	今日入院したマリー・アンダーソンの夫ですが，こちらの病院では付添いは必要ですか？	My wife, Mary Anderson, was admitted today. Is it necessary for me to stay the night?
看	いいえ，付き添う必要はありません．入院中は看護師がお世話をします．	That won't be necessary. Your wife will be cared for by the nursing staff while she is here.
家	わかりました．でも，妻の様子が心配なので，今夜は付添いたいのですが，いいですか？	I see. However, I am worried about my wife's condition. Is it OK for me to stay the night with her?
看	はい，どうぞ．でも，この病院では付添には医師の許可が必要です．病院のきまりでは，家族付添許可申請書を提出して頂くことになっています．今お持ちしますので，しばらくお待ち下さい．	Yes, you may. However, according to the hospital regulations, you will need her doctor's OK to stay overnight. There is a form you will have to fill out. Please wait here and I will bring one to you.
家	よろしくお願いします．	Thank you so much.
	…………	…………
看	これがその書類です．ご記入	Here it is. After you are finished

の上，ナースステーションまでお持ち下さい．	filling it out, please bring it to the nurses' station.
家 はい，すぐに書きます．	OK, I will do it right away.
看 付添の方の寝具は1日300円でお貸ししています．どうなさいますか？	There will be a 300 yen a day charge for bedding, if you need it. What do you think?
家 ええ，お願いします．	Yes, I will need some bedding. Thank you.
看 では，手配をします．あとで業者がお部屋にお届けしますので，そこで代金をお支払い下さい．	Alright, I will make the necessary arrangements. When the bed arrives, please pay the delivery person.
家 はい，わかりました．	Will do.

▶ Optional Vocabulary

ひと晩付き添う　stay the night, stay overnight, spend the night／
病院のきまり　hospital regulations, hospital rules

18

退　院
Hospital Discharge

退院準備
Getting Ready to Return Home

Track 47

看	グレイさん，3日後に退院できるそうですね(⇨ **OP**).	Hello Mr. Gray, **in three days you'll be able to leave us**.
患	ええ．今日，平野先生がそう言っていました．ようやく我が家に帰れます．	Yep. Dr. Hirano said the same thing earlier. I can't wait to get home.
看	本当に良かったですね．退院後のご自宅での生活について，ご家族にも説明させて頂きたいのですが，今日はどなたか来られる予定ですか？	I am happy for you, too. I would like to explain a few things to a family member about your lifestyle changes after you're discharged. Is anyone planning on visiting you today? (⇨ Eric's Tip 23)
患	はい．妻が昼過ぎに来ると言っていました．	Yeah, my wife said she would be here after lunch.
看	それでは，今日の午後に説明させて頂いてよろしいでしょうか．	So, it will be OK for me to talk to her this afternoon?
患	ええ．ぜひお願いします．	Yes, please do so.
看	では，奥様がおいでになられたらお知らせ下さい．	When she arrives, please let me know.
患	はい．そうします．	Sure, will do.

Optional Phrases

◘ …3日後に退院できるそうですね．
- …in three days you'll be able to leave us.
- …in three days you'll be able to go home.
- …in three days you'll be discharged.

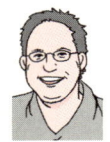

> **Eric's Tip 23　質問には some も OK**
> 疑問文に some を使うことは，文法的には正しくないのですが，ネイティブスピーカーはとてもよく使います．"Is anyone planning on visiting you today?" よりも，"Is someone planning on visiting you today?" の方が自然です．会話中の質問での some と any の区別は，気にするほどのことではありません．

退院時の心配事
Concerns about Being Discharged

Track 48

看　明日は退院ですね．家に帰ってからのことで，何かご心配はありませんか．
You will be discharged tomorrow. Do you have any concerns about returning home?

患　ええ，動くとすぐに息切れするので，以前のように家事ができないことが困ります．
Yeah, when I move I am soon out of breath. I won't be able to do housework like before and that's going to be a problem.

看 ご心配ですね．時々休みながら，無理をしない程度に動く必要がありますね．体を少しずつ慣らしていきましょう．	I see your point. You're going to have rest from time to time and not strain yourself. Your strength will return slowly but surely.
患 ええ，そうですね．	Yes, I hope so.
看 昨日，ご主人と娘さんにお話したのですが，しばらくの間，家事はお二人で分担すると言っておられましたよ．	Yesterday, I spoke with your husband and daughter and they said they would help out with the chores.
患 ええ，そう言ってはくれるのですが，二人ともほとんど家事をしたことがないのです．それに娘はまだ中学生ですから．	Yes, I know they said that, but they have never really helped me around the house. My daughter is still in junior high.
看 ご心配なお気持ちはよくわかります．でも，少し任せてみてはいかがですか？ 娘さんにもいい経験になると思いますよ．	I really understand your worries. But, if you give her a little responsibility, she should be OK. I think it will be good for your daughter.
患 そうですね．そうなることを願いましょう．ところで，退院の時間はいつでもいいのでしょうか？	That's right. I surely hope so. By the way, may I leave anytime tomorrow?
看 入院待機の方がおられるので，午前11時までにお願いします．	Since we have patients waiting to be admitted, we would appreciate it if you left before 11 AM.
患 わかりました．お話できてよかったです．	I see. I am really glad we were able to talk.

IV

周 手 術 期

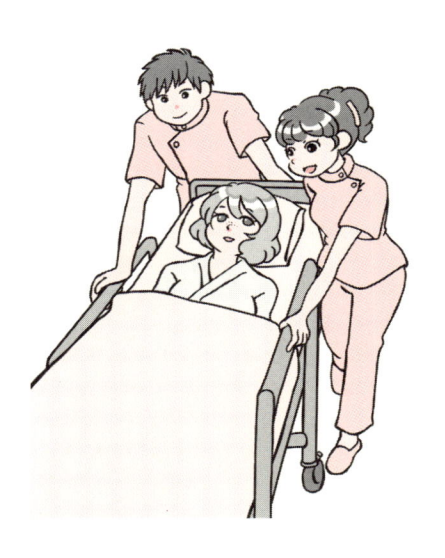

19

手 術 前
Before Surgery

術前オリエンテーション
Preoperative Guidance

Track 49

看	ブレアさん，山田医師からの手術についての説明と，大田医師からの麻酔についての説明は理解できましたか？	Hello, Mr. Blair, I take it that you understood what Dr. Yamada and Dr. Ohta said about your upcoming surgery and anesthesia?
患	ええ，大丈夫です．とてもわかりやすく説明して頂けましたし，質問にも答えて頂けました．	Yes, I did. Their explanations were very easy to follow, and they answered all of my questions.
看	それは良かったです．今から，手術に向けた準備について説明させて頂いてもよろしいでしょうか？	I am glad to hear that. Now I am going to talk about what we will do to prepare for your surgery. Is that OK?
患	はい，もちろん．	Yes, of course.
看	ブレアさんは，米国の病院でも手術を受けたことがあるとお伺いしています．	According to your records, you have undergone a surgery in America.
患	ええ，5年前に胆石の手術を受けました．	Yes, five years ago, I had some gallstones removed.
看	そのときに何か困ったことはありましたか？	At that time, did you experience any complications?

19. 手 術 前

患 いいえ，全く．その日のうちに家に帰れましたし，3日後には仕事に行くこともできました．	Nope, none at all. I went home the same day, and three days later I was back at work.
看 そうでしたか．今回はもう少し時間のかかる大きな手術ですので，万全な準備が必要になります．	Is that right? This time, however, your surgery is going to be more complex, so we are going to need more thorough preparations.
患 ええ，わかります．	OK, I see.

▶ Optional Vocabulary

術 前　pre-op 常, preoperative 医

▶ Additional Vocabulary

日帰り手術　day surgery 常, outpatient basis 常, ambulatory surgery 医／　内視鏡的手術　endoscopic operation, endoscopic surgery／　試験開腹　exploratory surgery／　侵襲的手術　invasive surgery／　最小侵襲手術　minimal invasive surgery／　低侵襲手術　minimally invasive surgery／　非侵襲的手術　non invasive surgery／　生 検　biopsy

手術に必要なもの
Things to Prepare for Surgery

Track 50

看 ブレアさん，これは手術前に準備しておいて頂くもののリストです．	Mr. Blair, here is a list of everything you will need after your surgery. Please get them ready a day before.
患 どれどれ．"ゆかた"と"T字帯"ですか？	Let me see. Why do I need a "yukata" and a "loincloth"?
看 ええ，手術の後はしばらく思うように動けないので，こういったものであれば，着替えが簡単にできます．それに，お腹に傷ができますから，傷に当たるような衣類はしばらく着ない方が良いのです．	Well, after your surgery it will be difficult for you to move for some time. As such, the yukata and loincloth will be easy to change. Besides, you are going to have an incision on your abdomen, and wearing loose clothing is preferable.
患 全く新しい体験になりそうです．	All this is new to me.
看 日本人でも手術でも受けない限り，着ることはないと思います．	Actually, if people in Japan don't have surgery, this will be new to them, too.
患 "吸い飲み"もしくは"ストロー付きカップ"ですか？赤ちゃん用品みたいですね．(⇨ **Eric's Tip 24**)	Why do I need a "suinomi" or a "cup with a built-in straw"? It sounds like something for a baby.
看 確かに，そうですね．でもこういった物があれば，起き上がらなくても，寝たままの状態で水が飲めます．	That's so, but it will allow you to drink even while lying flat on your back.
患 それは便利ですね．どういった店で購入すればいいのでしょうか？	That's convenient. Can you tell me where I can buy these things?

看 ご心配なく．全部，院内の売店で買えます．　　Don't worry. We sell everything here in the hospital.

患 では，今日中に買っておきます．　　OK, I will go buy the stuff today.

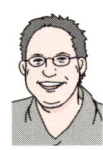

Eric's Tip 24　欧米の男性はストローを使わない?!
欧米の男性はストローを使うのは女性と子供だというイメージをもっているので，使いたくないという患者さんもいるかもしれません．

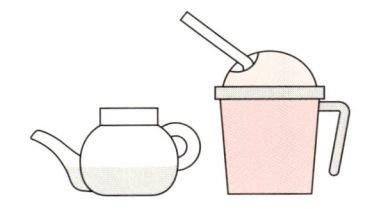

手術前の準備
Pre-op Preparations

Track 51

看 エバンスさんの手術は，4日後，3月8日月曜日9時からの予定です．麻酔は全身麻酔で行います．	Ms. Evans, you are scheduled to have your surgery four days from now on Monday, March 8th, at 9 AM. You will be under general anesthesia.
患 はい，新井先生から伺っています．	Yes, that's what Dr. Arai told me.
看 風邪をひくと**手術が延期になることがあります**(⇨ **OP**)ので，手洗いやうがいをこまめにして下さい．	If you catch a cold, **we will have to postpone your surgery**, so please be sure to wash your hands and gargle regularly.*
患 延期になったら困るので，気をつけます．	Postponing the surgery would be a real pain in the neck, I will be sure to do so.
看 手術前日の予定を確認しておきましょう．まず，手術後，しばらく入浴できなくなるので，手術前日は，体と髪をよく洗っておいて下さい．爪も切っておきましょう．	Now, let's go over what will happen the day before your surgery. First, after your surgery, you won't be able to bathe for a while. Therefore, the day before your surgery be sure to bathe and wash your hair. Cut your fingernails also.
患 はい，わかりました．	Yes, I see.
看 夕食以降は何も食べないで下さい．でも，飲水は深夜12時まで可能です．	After dinner that day, you won't be able to eat anything. However, you can drink water until midnight.
患 わかりました．	I understand.
看 夜9時ごろ，下剤と安定剤を	At around 9 PM, we will give

---

* おぼえておきたい表現 **4** (p.112)参照．

	内服して頂きます.	you a laxative and a sedative.
患	下剤ですか?	A laxative?
看	ええ,手術に向けて腸を空っぽにしておく必要があります(⇨ OP). 手術当日の朝6時ごろ,浣腸もします.	Yes. **Before your surgery, it's necessary to have an empty GI* tract.** On the morning of your surgery around 6 AM, we will also give you an enema.
患	"それはどうも".	Lucky me(⇨ **Eric's Tip 25**).

▶ Optional Vocabulary

手 術　surgery 常, operation 常, procedure 医

Optional Phrases

❏ …手術が延期になることがあります.	...we will have to postpone your surgery. ...we will have to reschedule your surgery. ...we will have to delay your surgery. ...we will have to put off your surgery.
❏ …手術に向けて腸を空っぽにしておく必要があります.	...before your surgery, it's necessary to have an empty GI tract. ...before your surgery, it's necessary to have an empty stomach(⇨ **Shigemi's Tip 2**). ...before your surgery, it's necessary to have you cleaned out.　(丁寧ではない表現)

---

* GI: gastrointestinal

▶ Additional Vocabulary

全身麻酔　general anesthesia ／　局所麻酔　local anesthesia ／
局所（局部）麻酔　regional anesthesia

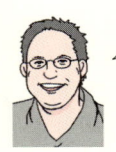

> **Eric's Tip 25**　皮肉なジョークは聞き流しましょう
> 患者さんによっては"Lucky me.", "It's going to be fun."のように，ジョークや皮肉を言うかもしれません．本当に"良かった．ついてる．", "それは楽しみですね．"と思っているわけではありません．ストレス解消の独り言だと思って，特に返事をする必要もなく，聞き流して大丈夫です．

> **Shigemi's Tip 2**　"Stomach"で通じます
> 洗腸の説明にわざわざ"intestine（腸）"という言葉を使わなくても"stomach（胃）"と言えば通じます．

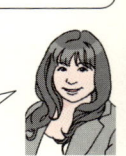

おぼえておきたい表現
4 頻度の表し方

頻度を表す単語はたくさんありますが，人によってその意味が違うことがあります．一般的にはこのような程度を表しています．

頻度スケール（Frequency scale）

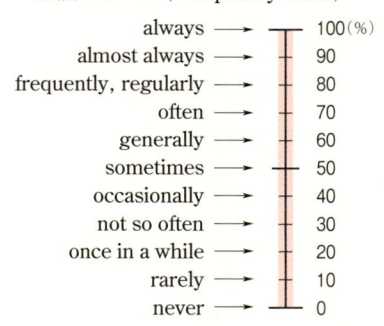

語	%
always	100 (%)
almost always	90
frequently, regularly	80
often	70
generally	60
sometimes	50
occasionally	40
not so often	30
once in a while	20
rarely	10
never	0

手術当日の準備
Day of Surgery Preparations

Track 52

看 エバンスさん，では次に，手術当日の予定を確認しておきましょう．朝6時の浣腸後は，排便があったかどうかを看護師に知らせて下さい（⇨ **OP**）．

Now Ms. Evans, let's go over the day of your surgery. **After your enema** at 6 AM, **please let us know if it had any effect.**

患 ええ，お知らせします．

OK, I will be sure to tell you.

看 朝8時までに，トイレを済ませて手術着に着替えて頂きます．そのとき，眼鏡，コンタクトレンズ，入歯，指輪，時計，かつらなど，身に付けているものは全て外して下さい．

By 8 AM, be sure to finish going to the bathroom and change into your surgical gown. At that time, be sure to remove your glasses, contacts, dentures, rings, watch, wig, etc…basically anything on your body.

患 はい，わかりました．

OK, I understand.

看 8時に麻酔の導入がスムーズにいくように鎮静剤を注射します．

At 8 AM, to help with your anesthesia, we will administer a sedative.

患 注射があるのですね．

You are going to use a needle?

看 ええ．その後，ストレッチャーに乗って，8時20分に手術室に移動します．

Yes, I am afraid so. After that, we will lie you down on a stretcher and transfer you to the operating room at 8:20.

患 出発は8時20分ですね．

The fun starts at 8:20?

看 ええ，そうです．ご家族は当日，病院においでになりますか？

That's right. Will anyone from your family be here that morning?

患 夫と娘が来てくれることになっています．

Yes, my husband and daughter will be here.

看 そうですか．8時までに来て頂いて下さい．手術の間は，手術室横の部屋でお待ち頂くことをお伝え下さい．	Is that so? Make sure they are here before 8 AM. And tell them that they can wait in the room next to the operating room.
患 ええ，伝えます．	OK, I will.
看 何か，わからないことがありましたら，いつでもお知らせ下さい．	If you have any questions, please feel free to ask anytime.
患 はい，ありがとうございます．	Yes, thank you very much.

▶ Optional Vocabulary

コンタクトレンズ　contacts, contact lenses ／　手術室　operating room (OR)常, surgery room常, operating suite常, operating theater医

Optional Phrases

◘ 浣腸後は，排便があったかどうかを看護師に知らせて下さい．	After your enema, please let us know if it had any effect.
	After your enema, please let us know if it worked or not.
	After your enema, please let us know if it made you go.
	After your enema, please let us know if anything came out.

手術室看護師の術前訪問
Pre-op Visit by OR Nurse

Track 53

看	スコットさん,こんにちは.はじめまして.	Hello Mr. Scott, nice to meet you.
患	こちらこそ.	Likewise.
看	スコットさんの手術を担当させて頂く看護師の小川です.	My name is Ogawa and I will be your OR nurse.
患	手術室でお世話になるのですね.	So you will be with me in the operating room?
看	ええ.少しお話しさせて頂いてもよろしいでしょうか?	Yes, I will. May I talk to you about a few things?
患	はい,どうぞ.	Sure, go ahead.
看	初めての手術だと伺っています.ご心配なことはありませんか?(⇨ OP)	I heard this will be your first surgery ever. **Are you worried about anything**?*
患	ええ,たくさんあります.(⇨ Eric's Tip 26)	You bet I am.
看	たとえば?	For example?
患	手術室自体が想像できないので,なんだか怖い感じです.	First, I can't imagine what the operating room will look like, which is kind of disturbing.
看	よろしければ,手術室を見学してみませんか?(⇨ OP) 事前に見ておくことで,安心したと多くの患者さんが言っておられます.	**If you would like, I can give you a tour of the** OR. Many patients have told me that such a tour helped. What do you think?
患	ぜひ,私にも見学させて下さい.	Sure, I would appreciate that.

---

* afraid of, scared of, fear of (怖い,恐怖を感じる) には"弱虫"というネガティブなイメージが付きまとうため,欧米人の特に成人男性は使わない表現です. anxious, worried, concerned (心配) の方がよく使われます.

看 では早速，今日の午後 2 時過ぎはいかがですか？ スコットさんの今日の検査はそれまでには全て終わっていると病棟の看護師に聞いています．	Alright, how about today a little after 2 PM? I heard from a nurse on this floor that you will be finished with your tests by that time.
患 ああそうですか．	Is that so?
看 では 2 時にお迎えに参ります．	I will be back around 2 PM.
患 よろしくお願いします．	See you then.

Optional Phrases

◘ ご心配なことはありませんか？	Are you worried about anything? Do you have any concerns? Is there anything worrying you? Are you anxious about anything?
◘ よろしければ，～を見学してみませんか？	If you would like, I can give you a tour of the ～. If you want, I can give you a tour of the ～. If you would like, I can show you around the ～. If you are interested, would you like a tour of the ～.

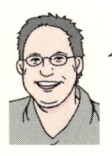

Eric's Tip 26　日本の医療に不安を抱く外国人もいる

日本の病院で受ける手術には，不安を抱いている外国人が多いようです．医療システムが自国と違うという理由だけでなく，残念ながら日本の病院では医療ミスが多いというイメージをもっていると思われます．

手術後の呼吸方法
Post-op Breathing Techniques

Track 54

看 手術後に困らないように，呼吸訓練をしておきましょう．	To help make things easier for you post-op, let's practice some breathing techniques.
患 特別な呼吸法が必要なのですか？	Will it be necessary for me to breathe in a special way?
看 特別というわけでもないのですが，手術後は寝た状態で，傷の痛みもあるので，練習しておくと安心です．まずは，深呼吸してみましょう．	It's not a special way, but after your surgery you will be lying on your back and may be in pain, therefore, it's better to practice now. First, let's take a deep breath.
患 こんな感じですか．	Like this?
看 ええ，そうです．とても上手に腹式呼吸ができていますね．	That's right. Wow, you are very good at breathing from your abdomen.
患 そうですか？ 特に意識はしていないのですが．	Is that so? I guess it comes naturally.
看 手術後は呼吸が浅くなりがちです．術後合併症の肺炎を予防するために，ときどきは深呼吸することが大切です．	After your surgery, you will tend to take shallow breaths. It will be important for you to take deep breaths sometimes to help prevent post-op pneumonia complications.
患 それはどうも，勉強になりました．	Thank you, I learned something new today.
看 手をこんなふうに下腹部の上において，息を吸ったときにお腹が膨らむのを確認してみましょう．	Now place your hands on your lower abdomen, like this. (⇨ **Shigemi's Tip 3**) When you inhale, be sure that your abdomen expands, like this.

| 患 | はい，膨らんでいます． | Yes, I can feel it. |
| 看 | 口からゆっくりと息を吐きましょう．鼻から息を吸って，お腹を膨らませて下さい．そうです．**良い感じです**(⇨ **OP**). | Be sure to exhale slowly from your mouth. Then inhale through your nose, and your abdomen will expand. That's right, **you are doing great**. |

Optional Phrases

◘ 良い感じです．　　　You are doing great.　　　より丁寧
　　　　　　　　　　　Excellent job.　　　　　　　↑
　　　　　　　　　　　Wonderful.

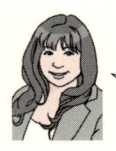

Shigemi's Tip 3　百聞は一見にしかず
動作などを英語で説明する場合，"like this"と言って，実際にやって見せる方がよいでしょう．

おぼえておきたい表現
5 ほめ言葉の程度 (Praise Strength)

ほめ言葉にはいろいろあります．愛のムチもときには必要ですが，ほめてもらうことを期待する人もたくさんいます．ただし，ほめすぎには注意しましょう．期待どおりにできていないときにはきちんと伝えましょう．

非常に素晴らしい．	Perfect.
	Fantastic.
	Excellent.
素晴らしい．	Great.
	Wonderful.
	Very good.
いいですね．	Good.
	Nice job.
	Good job.
まあまあです．	OK.
	So so.
	Fair.

手 術 当 日
Day of the Operation

手術室への移動
Transferring to the OR

Track 55

看 エバンスさん，30分後に手術室に入ります．トイレを済ませて手術着に着替えて，この帽子を付けて下さい．準備ができたらお知らせ下さい．	Mrs. Evans, we'll be taking you to the operating room in 30 minutes. After going to the bathroom one last time, please change into your operation gown and put this paper cap on your head. When you are ready, please let me know.
患 はい…着替えました．	Sure. OK, I have finished changing.
看 コンタクトレンズ，入歯，指輪，時計は外しましたか？	Have you removed your contacts, dentures, rings, and watch?
患 そういえば指輪がまだでした．両手にしているのですが，結婚指輪は付けていてもいいですか？	Now that you mention it, I forgot to take off my rings. I have rings on both hands. Can I keep my wedding ring on?
看 シンプルな結婚指輪であれば，付けたままでも大丈夫です．飾りの付いた指輪は外して，ご家族に預けておきま	If it is a simple ring, you may keep it on. However, please remove flashy rings with stones. Could you please leave

しょう.	your other rings with a family member?
患 はい,そうします.	Yes, I will.
看 では,こちらのストレッチャーに寝て下さい.鎮静剤を注射しましょう.	Now, please lie down on this stretcher. You will be administered an anesthetic.
患 はい.	I see.
看 少しチクッとします.右手はしびれていませんか?	You will feel a little sting. Do you feel a tingling sensation in your right hand?
患 大丈夫です.	No, I am OK.
看 終わりです.軽くもんでおきましょう.	There, that's all. Let me rub the spot gently.
患 すぐに眠くなりますか?	Will I fall asleep soon?
看 いいえ,少しずつ効いてきますから,楽にしていて下さい.では手術室に行きましょう.ご家族の皆さんも一緒にどうぞ.お待ち頂く場所までご案内します.	No, you will feel the effects slowly, please try to relax. OK, now let's get you to the OR. Your family may join us. I will show them the waiting room.

▶ Optional Vocabulary

(結婚)指輪　(wedding) ring 囡, (wedding) band 男

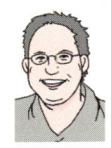

Eric's Tip 27　結婚指輪は外せない!
欧米人は,結婚指輪に特別な意味を感じている人も多いので,外すことを嫌がるかもしれません.

Shigemi's Tip 4　ゆるい指輪はテープで固定!
日本では手術や検査のときに指輪を外してもらうのが当然ですが,米国では,手術の妨げにならない限り,シンプルな結婚指輪は付けたままでも OK でした.ゆるくて外れそうな指輪は,テープを貼って止めておきましょう.

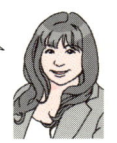

手術室での会話
A Conversation in the OR

Track 56

看 スコットさん，おはようございます．先日お目にかかった小川です．	Good morning, Mr. Scott. We met the other day. My name is Ogawa.
患 またお会いできましたね．	That's right. Nice to see you again.
看 ご気分はいかがですか？	How are you feeling today?
患 少し眠いです．	I'm a little sleepy.
看 **寒くはないですか？**(⇨ OP)	**Are you cold at all?**
患 大丈夫です．	No, I'm fine. Thanks.
看 **手術前の準備を始めます**(⇨ OP)．寒く感じたらいつでも言って下さい．	**We are going to start prepping you for surgery.** If you feel cold, please feel free to let us know.
患 はい，わかりました．	Yes, I understand.
看 まず，左腕に自動血圧計を巻きましょう．手術中は血圧を定期的に測定します．これは心電図をモニターするためのシールで，胸に貼ります．	First, I will attach this automatic blood pressure cuff to your left arm. During your surgery, it will check your pressure from time to time. Now, I will attach these seals to your chest. They will help monitor your heart.
患 はい．	I see.
看 次に，右腕に点滴注射をしましょう．楽にしていて下さい．	Next, this IV will go into your right arm. Please try to relax.
患 はい．	OK.
看 最後に，足に血栓ができないように，両足に空気マッサージ器を付けましょう．大丈夫ですか？	Lastly, I will attach this air massager to your legs to help prevent blood clots. How do you feel?

20. 手 術 当 日

患 はい,問題ありません.　　　I'm fine. There are no problems.

Optional Phrases

- 寒くはないですか？
  - Are you cold at all?
  - Do you feel a chill?
  - Are you chilly at all?
  - Are you warm enough?

- 手術前の準備を始めます.
  - We are going to start prepping you for surgery. (一番自然な表現)
  - We are going to start preparing you for surgery.
  - We are going to start getting you ready for surgery.

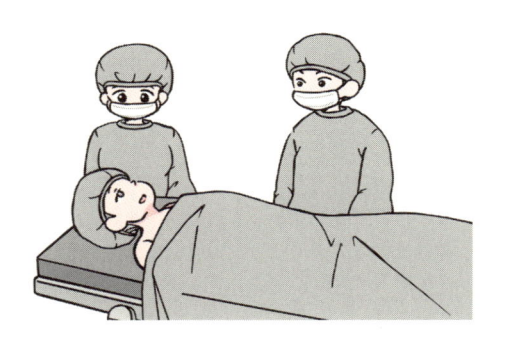

手術中の家族への説明
Talking to the Family of a Patient Mid-operation Track 57

看	ロマノさんのご家族はいらっしゃいますか？	Is the family of Mrs. Romano here?
家	はい，ここです．夫のジョニーです．これは娘のリサです．	Yes, we're over here. I am her husband, Johnny. And this is our daughter Lisa.
看	はじめまして．手術室の看護師の山田夕子です．**手術中の奥様の様子を伝えに来ました**（⇨ **OP**）．手術は今のところ順調に進んでいますので，どうぞご安心下さい（⇨ **Shigemi's Tip 5**）．	Nice to meet you. My name is Yuko Yamada and I am the OR nurse. **I came to let you know how your wife is doing.** Everything is going well so far, so please don't worry.
家	そうですか，それはよかった．悪性の腫瘍ではなかったのでしょうか？	Is that so? We are relieved to hear the good news! Was the tumor a malignant one?
看	それについては検査中なのでわかりません．検査結果は手術のあとに担当の川崎医師がご説明いたします．	I can't say for sure as we are running tests on it. When the operation is over, Dr. Kawasaki will come and share the results with you.
家	そうですか．じゃあ待ちます．	Is that right? We will wait until then.
看	手術はあと1時間くらいかかりそうです．昼食時間ですので，よろしければカフェテリアに行って食事をおとり下さい．	Your wife's surgery will probably take another hour. It is now lunch time, why don't you go get something to eat in the cafeteria?
家	そうですね．お腹も空いてきましたし．	Sounds good. We are kind of hungry.
看	何かありましたらお知らせし	Just in case there is some more

ますので,おひとりはここでお待ち下さい.	news, I recommend that one of you stay here though.
家 はい.娘が食事に行く間,私がここにいます.	OK. My daughter will go eat, while I stay here.

▶ Additional Vocabulary

悪性 malignant ／ 良性 benign (non-malignant)

Optional Phrases

◘ 手術中の奥様の様子を伝えに来ました.	I came to let you know how your wife is doing. I came to inform you on how your wife is doing. I am here to tell you how your wife is doing.

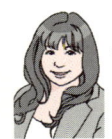

Shigemi's Tip 5　手術を待つ家族へのケア

日本では"何かあればお知らせします"と,手術中の待機を家族にお願いしますが,何もなくても家族は心配です.欧米では手術中の家族へのケアは看護師の役割として重視されています.

21 手術後
After Surgery

手術が終わって
After the Operation

CD Track 58

看	トーマスさん，手術が終わりましたよ．	Mr. Thomas, your operation's done.
患	えっ，もう？ 今，何時ですか？	What? Already? What time is it?
看	午後4時です．	It's 4 PM.
患	4時間も経ったのですか．手術は成功ですか？	I've been out for four hours? Was the operation a success?
看	はい，予定どおりです（⇨ **OP**）	Yes, **it went very smoothly**.
患	それはよかった．	That's good.
看	よく頑張りましたね．どこか痛いところはありませんか？	You did very well, indeed. Do you feel any pain right now?
患	喉が少し．	My throat hurts a little.
看	そうですか．喉に管が入っていたので，しばらく痛むかもしれません．	Is that so? You were intubated and your throat will be a little sore for a while.
患	じゃあ仕方ないですね．	Lucky me.
看	深呼吸をしてみてください．	Can you take a deep breath for me?
患	（深呼吸）	(Inhales deeply.)
看	はい，よくできています．吐き気はありませんか？	Very good! Well done! Do you feel nauseous at all?

21. 手術後

患	ありません.	Nope.
看	私の手をグーッと握ってみて下さい.	Can you squeeze my hand?
患	こうですか？	Like this?
看	はい, 結構です. 今度は足を動かしてみてください.	Yes, that's fine. Now can you move your feet for me?
患	こうですか？	Like this?
看	はい, 結構です. しびれや違和感はありませんか？(⇨ OP)	Yes, very good. **Do you feel numb or something is unusual**?
患	大丈夫です.	No, I am fine.
看	では, これから病室に戻りましょう. ご家族が待っていますよ. 酸素マスクをしばらく付けておきましょう.	Then let's get you back to your room. Your family is waiting for you. Let's put this oxygen mask on you for the time being.

Optional Phrases

◘ 予定どおりです.

Everything went according to schedule.　より丁寧

Everything went according to plan.

It went very smoothly.

There were no surprises.

丁寧さ

◘ しびれや違和感はありませんか？

Do you feel numb or something is unusual?　より丁寧

Do you feel numb or unpleasant?

Do you feel numb or something is strange?

Do you feel numb or out of wack?

丁寧さ

術後訪問
Post Surgery Visit

CD Track 59

看	スコットさん，こんにちは．手術を担当させて頂いた小川です．	Hello, Mr. Scott. I am Ogawa, your OR nurse.
患	またあなたですか？	It's you again. (⇨ Eric's Tip 28)
看	手術室についての感想をお聞きしたいのですが，よろしいでしょうか？	Do you mind if I ask some questions about your OR experience?
患	ええ，もちろん．	No, not at all.
看	手術前に説明にお伺いしましたが，お役に立ちましたか？	Did you find the explanation before your operation useful?
患	手術室についてイメージすることができました．顔を知っている看護師が手術を担当してくれるのは心強く感じました．	First, it was nice to imagine what the OR would be like. It also helped to see a face I knew in the OR.
看	それは良かったです．手術室がイメージと違っていたことはありますか？	I'm happy to hear that. Did anything surprise you in the OR?
患	思っていたよりも明るい感じでした．	It was much brighter than I expected.
看	そうおっしゃる方が多いです．麻酔がかかるまでは，どんな感じでしたか？(⇨ **OP**)	Many people say the same thing. **Until the anesthetic took effect, how were you feeling?**
患	もう任せるしかないと思いました．麻酔がかかるまで看護師が手を握っていてくれたのは嬉しかったです．	I was at your mercy. I am happy that I was able to hold someone's hand while I was waiting to lose consciousness.
看	お役に立てて，私たちも嬉しいです．手術室の温度はどう	We are happy you are happy. How was the temperature in

	でしたか？	the OR?
患	ちょっと寒かったです．	It was a little cold.
看	それは申しわけありませんでした．気をつけるようにします．物音や会話で気になることはありませんでしたか？	Sorry about that. We'll be careful about that in the future. Were you bothered by anything you heard in the OR?
患	いえ，特にありません．	Not really.
看	よかったです．	That's good.

Optional Phrases

◘ 麻酔がかかるまでは，どんな感じでしたか？

Until the anesthetic took effect, how were you feeling?

Until the drugs took effect, how were you feeling?

Until the anesthetic kicked in, how did you feel?

Until the drugs kicked in, how did you feel?

より丁寧 ↑ 丁寧さ

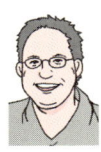

Eric's Tip 28　ネバー・ギブ・アップ！

会いたくない人に会ったとき，"It's you again." "I see we meet again." "Go away." "Leave me alone." などと機嫌の悪い患者さんは言うかもしれませんが，その言葉どおりの意味ではないので，優しく接しましょう．

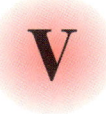

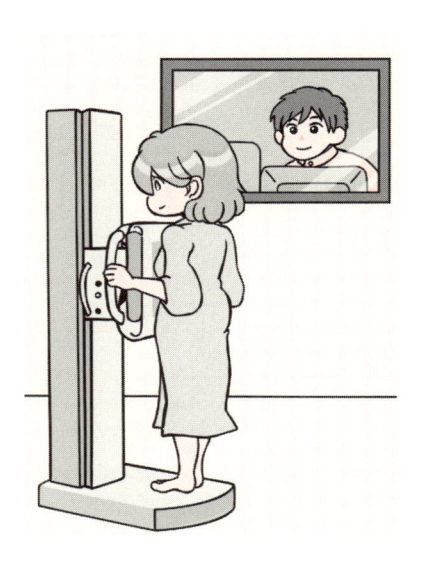

V

検　　　　査

22

検　査
Testing

血液検査
Blood Test

Track 60

看	こんにちは．確認のために，お名前を言って頂けますか？（⇨ **OP**）	Good afternoon. **First, may I have your name**? (⇨ Eric's Tip 29)
患	ナンシー・モリスです．	My name is Nancy Morris.
看	今日は3種類の血液検査があります．検査してもよろしいですか？	Today we are going to run three kinds of blood tests on you. Is that OK?
患	はい，先生がそう言っていました．	Sure. That's what my doctor told me.
看	以前に採血をして気分が悪くなったことはありませんか？（⇨ **OP**）	When your blood was taken in the past, **did you ever feel bad**?
患	いいえ，ありません．	Nope, never.
看	アルコール過敏症ですか？（⇨ **OP**）	**Are you allergic to** alcohol?
患	ええ，実はそうです．以前，予防注射のときに皮膚がただれてしまったことがあります．	Actually, I am. In the past, when I got an immunization shot, my skin got a rash.
看	では別の消毒薬を使いましょう．	OK. I'll use a different antiseptic then.

22. 検　査

患	聞いて頂いてよかったです！すっかり忘れていました．	I'm glad you asked!　I had completely forgotten about my allergy.
看	採血する腕のシャツの袖をまくって下さい．	Please roll up your sleeve, and I will take your blood.
患	これくらいでいいですか？	How's this?
看	はい大丈夫です．では駆血帯を巻きます．	That's just right.　Now I'm going to put a tourniquet around your upper arm.
患	はい．	OK.
看	親指を中にして軽く握って下さい(⇨ **OP**)．消毒をします．それではチクリとします．	**Please make a ball with your fist**.　Now, I'll sterilize the area.　This may sting a little.
患	痛っ．	Ouch.
看	はい，終了です．手を楽にして下さい．もまないで，5分くらい指でしっかり押さえて圧迫して下さい．出血が止まったら，この絆創膏を貼って下さい．この後は，こちら側の腕で重いものは持たないようにして下さい．	Alright, we're finished.　Please relax your hand.　Don't rub it, and please apply pressure here with a finger for about five minutes.　Once the bleeding has stopped, put this bandage over it.　By the way, please avoid lifting heavy things with this arm.
患	はい，わかりました．	I see.

▶ Optional Vocabulary

過敏症　allergy 常, sensitivity 医 ／　～過敏症である　be allergic to ～常, have a/an ～ allergy 常, be sensitive to ～医, have a/an ～ sensitivity 医 ／　消毒薬　antiseptic, cleaner, disinfectant, bactericide 医

Optional Phrases

- 確認のために，お名前を言って頂けますか？

  First, may I confirm your name?
  First, may I have your name?
  First, can I have your name?
  First, please tell me your name.

  より丁寧 ↑ 丁寧さ

- 以前に気分が悪くなったことはありませんか？

  Did you ever feel like you wanted to die?
  Did you ever feel terrible?
  Did you ever feel awful?
  Did you ever feel bad?
  Did you ever feel funny?

  より悪い ↑ 気分の悪さ

- 〜過敏症ですか？

  Do you have a/an 〜 allergy?
  Do you have a/an 〜 sensitivity?
  Are you allergic to 〜?
  Are you sensitive to 〜?

- 親指を中にして軽く握って下さい．

  Please make a ball with your fist.
  Please make a fist.

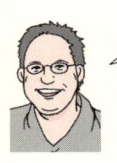

Eric's Tip 29　手順をふむときには First から

"First, ..." は「まず〜」という感じで，いくつかの手順がある際に，一番最初に使ってみましょう．そうすれば患者さんは，次には何かがある，ということを予測して心づもりもしやすくなります．

尿 検 査
Urine Test

Track 61

看	ジョーンズさん，尿検査の指示が出ていますが，聞いていますか？	Mr. Jones, you were told to have a urine test, is that correct?
患	はい，伺っています．	That's right.
看	今から排尿できますか？(⇒ OP)	**Will you be able to go now?**
患	はい，たぶん．	I think so.
看	では，このコップをお持ちになって，検査室横のトイレにお入り下さい．最初に少しだけトイレに排尿した後で，中間尿をコップの3分の1*まで採って下さい．検体の入ったコップは，トイレ内の台の上に置いておいて下さい．	OK, now take this cup with you into the toilet next to this testing room. At first, urinate a little into the toilet. Midstream, pee into the cup until it is one third filled. Please leave the cup on the tray in the toilet.
患	用が済んだことを誰かにお知らせした方がいいですか？	When I am done, who should I tell?
看	その必要はありません．	That won't be necessary.
患	わかりました．	I see.

▶ Optional Vocabulary

尿 number one 常，pee pee 幼，pee 幼，urine 医／ 排 尿 go number one 常，go pee pee 幼，go pee 幼，urinate 医／ トイレ toilet 常，restroom 常，bathroom 常，little boy's room 幼，little girl's room 幼，men's room 男，ladies room 女

---

* おぼえておきたい表現 6 (p.136)参照．

Optional Phrases

◘ 今から排尿できますか？

Will you be able to urinate now?
Will you be able to go now?
Can you go now?
Can you fill this cup?

より丁寧 ↑ 丁寧さ

おぼえておきたい表現
6 分数の読み方

分数は一般的には分子を序数で先に読み，分母を序数で後に読みます．たとえば，3分の1(1/3)は，one third と読みますが，a third でも大丈夫です．

1/2	2分の1	half
1/3	3分の1	one third（あるいは a third）
2/3	3分の2	two thirds
1/4	4分の1	one fourth（a quarter の方が自然）
3/4	4分の3	three fourths
1/5	5分の1	one fifth
2/5	5分の2	two fifths
3/100	100分の3	three one-hundredths

血糖値検査
Blood Sugar Test

Track 62

看 ミラーさん，血糖値を調べますが，よろしいですか？

Mrs. Miller, we are now going to check your blood sugar level. Is that OK?

22. 検　査

患 腕からたくさん血液を採るのですか？	Are you going to take a lot of blood from my arm?
看 いいえ．指先からほんの1滴だけ下さい．	Actually, I just need a drop of blood from the tip of your finger.
患 指先から？　何だか痛そうですね．	The tip of my finger?　That sounds like it's gonna hurt.
看 たいしたことはありませんよ．チクッとするだけです．朝ごはんは何時に食べましたか？	It shouldn't hurt too much.　I am just going to prick your finger.　By the way, when did you eat breakfast?
患 7時半でした．	I ate at 7:30.
看 その後に何か召し上がりましたか？（⇨ **OP**）	**Have you had anything since?**
患 いいえ，何も食べていません．	No, nothing.
看 では3時間たっていますね．薬指を出して頂けますか．最初にアルコール綿で消毒してから，この器具で針を刺します．準備はいいですか？	Then it's been a full three hours.　Please give me your index finger.　I will first swab it with an antiseptic, then prick you with this.　Are you ready?
患 たぶん…．	Maybe...
看 もう刺しました．指を押して血液を1滴だけこの検査用紙に付けます．	We're done.　Please put a drop of blood onto this testing sheet.
患 意外と簡単ですね．	That was really simple!
看 血糖値は106 mg/dL です．	And your blood sugar level is 106 (one oh six).

Optional Phrases

◘ その後に何か召し上がりましたか？	Have you eaten anything since? Have you had anything since? Did you eat anything after that?

胸部レントゲン線検査
Taking a Chest X-ray

Track 63

看	モリスさん,レントゲン室1にお入り下さい.(⇨ OP)	Mrs. Morris, **please go to X-ray room number 1**.
患	はい.	Sure.
看	胸のレントゲンを撮ります.上半身だけ下着を脱いでTシャツ1枚になって下さい.Tシャツにボタンや金具がある場合は,このガウンに着替えて下さい.ネックレスは外しましょう.	We are going to take an X-ray of your chest. You may keep your pants/skirt on, but please strip down to your t-shirt. If you have buttons or metal on your t-shirt, please change into this gown. And please remove your necklace, too.
患	はい,わかりました.仕度ができました.	Yes, I understand. I am done.
看	髪が長いですね.このゴムバンドで上の方に束ねて頂けますか?	Your hair is quite long. Would you mind putting it up with this rubber band?
患	はい,これでいいですか.	OK, like this?
看	バッチリです.ではこちらに上って下さい.プロテクターを腰の後ろに受けましょう.	Perfect. Now, please stand on this. And let's put this protector around your waist.
患	はい.	OK.
看	あごをここに載せて,胸をここに密着させて下さい.肩には力を入れずに楽にしていて下さい.撮影のときは,深く息を吸って,そのまま息を止めましょう.	Put your chin here, please. And press your chest against here. Please relax your shoulders. When we take the X-ray, please take a deep breath and hold it.
患	はい.	I see.
技	大きく息を吸って下さい.そのまま止めて下さい.はい,	Take a deep breath, please. And hold it. OK, we're done.

22. 検　査

終わりです．楽にして下さい．	Please relax.
看 気分は悪くないですか？	How are you feeling?
患 大丈夫です．	I'm alright.
看 はい．では，着替えて，ホールで少しお待ち下さい．	Good. Now please change back into your clothes and wait in the hall.
患 そうします．	Will do.*

Optional Phrases

◘ レントゲン室1にお入り下さい．

① 検査室の中から呼ぶとき	Please enter X-ray room number 1.
② 検査室の前で呼ぶとき	Please come to X-ray room number 1.
③ 検査室の外で呼ぶとき	Please go to X-ray room number 1.

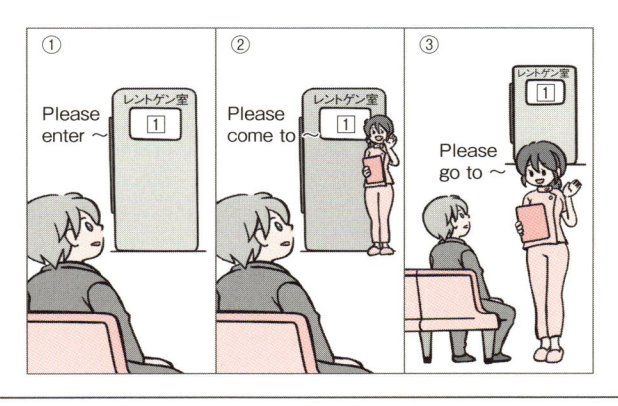

---

* "I will be sure to do so."の略で自然な言い方です．

CT 検査
CT Scan

Track 64

看 カーパーさん，こちらへどうぞ．足元に気をつけて，ここに寝て下さい．	Mr. Carper, please come this way. Please watch your step and lie down here.
患 はい．	OK.
看 今から点滴で造影剤を入れます．以前に造影剤で気分が悪くなったことはありませんか？	Now I am going to administer a contrast dye through this IV. In the past, when you received such a dye, did it make you feel sick?
患 造影剤を使った検査は受けたことがないと思います．	Actually, I think this is my first time to have a test with a contrast dye.
看 わかりました．造影剤が入ると体の中が熱く感じますが，心配ありません．でも，異常を感じたら，すぐに知らせて下さい．	I see. After I inject you with the dye, you are going to start feeling warm. Please don't worry about this. However, if you feel something is wrong, please let me know.
患 そうします．	I will.
看 検査が始まると，撮影台が動きます．「動かないで下さい」「息を止めて下さい」といった指示があったら，そのようにして下さい．	When the scan starts, the table will move. When the technician says, "Please don't move."and "Please don't breathe."be sure to follow her directions.
患 わかりました．	I see.
看 終わりです．お疲れさまでした（⇨ Eric's Tip 30）．台から降りて着替えましょう．	We're finished. Thank you for your cooperation. Feel free to come off the table and change back into your clothes.

22. 検　　査

患 はい．	OK.
看 造影剤を体から早く出すために，水分を多目に補給して下さい．しばらくしてから発疹が出ることもあります．その場合は，病院にご連絡下さい．	To get the contrast dye out of your body as quickly as possible, please drink a lot of water. If you break out into a rash, please contact us.
患 はい，そうします．	I will be sure to do so.

▶ Optional Vocabulary

造影剤　contrast dye 常, contrast agent 常, contrast medium 医, radiopaque dye 医

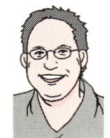

Eric's Tip 30　「お疲れさま」は直訳しない

日本では「お疲れさまでした」という表現をよく使いますが，英語にはそういう言葉かけはありませんので，"Thank you for your cooperation." と言ってみましょう．直訳の "You must be tired." には意味がありません．

上部消化管内視鏡検査
Upper Gastrointestinal (GI) Tract Endoscopy Track 65

患	こんにちは.10時に予約しているベーカーです.	Hello. My name is Baker. I have an appointment for 10 AM.
看	こんにちは,ベーカーさん.胃カメラ検査ですね.同意書と問診表(付録E, p.160)をお持ち頂けましたか?	Hello, Mr. Baker. You are here for a gastroscopy, aren't you? Do you have your consent form and questionnaire with you?
患	はい,これです.	Yep, here you go.
看	ありがとうございます.では検査室にお入り下さい.	Thank you. OK, please enter the examination room.
	....	....
	こちらへどうぞ.眼鏡は外しましょう.ズボンのベルトは緩めて下さい.上着やカバンはそこのかごに入れて下さい.	This way, please. Let's remove your glasses. Please loosen your belt a little. Your shirt and bag can go into this basket here.
患	はい.どれくらい時間がかかりますか?	OK. By the way, how long will this take?
看	準備も含めて30分以内です.昨夜から何も食べていませんね?	Including prep time, it'll take less than 30 minutes. You haven't eaten anything since last night, right?
患	はい,水を飲んだだけです.	That's right. I've only had some water.
看	**注意を守って下さってありがとうございます**(⇨ **OP**, Eric's Tip 31).今,ご気分はいかがですか?	**Thanks for following the instructions**. And how do you feel now?
患	特に問題ありません.	I'm fine.
看	わかりました.これは胃の中	I see. This medicine will

の泡を消す薬です．まずお飲み下さい．	dissolve the bubbles in your stomach. Please take it, first.
患 はい…美味しいものではありませんね．	OK...that's pretty bad.
看 ええ，申しわけありません．次に胃の動きを抑える注射を肩にします．	Yeah, sorry about that. Next, I will give you a shot in your upper arm to slow down the movement of your stomach.
患 はい．	OK.
看 胃カメラ検査中は，鼻でゆっくり呼吸しましょう．	During the gastroscopy, please breathe slowly through your nose.
患 はい，わかりました．	Yes, I will.
看 検査終了です．喉に麻酔をしていますので，約1時間は食べたり飲んだりしないで下さい．検査中，胃に空気を入れたので，お腹が張った感じがするかもしれませんが，しばらくすると消えます．もし何かありましたら，ご連絡下さい．	OK, we're done. It will take about an hour for the anesthetic to wear off. For the next hour, please don't eat or drink anything. During the exam, we put air into your stomach, so you probably feel bloated now. That will go away in a while. If you need anything, please feel free to contact us.
患 はい，ありがとうございました．	Yes, thank you very much.

Optional Phrases

◘ 注意を守って下さってありがとうございます.

- I appreciate your following our instructions.
- I appreciate your following our directions.
- Thanks for following the instructions.
- Thanks for following the directions.

より丁寧 ↑ 丁寧さ

Eric's Tip 31　患者さんはお客様？

米国では医療もビジネスなので，患者は顧客（customers）として扱われることを期待しています．また多くの患者が医療者の出す指示に従わないこと "noncompliance（ノンコンプライアンス）" や "nonadhearance（ノンアドヒアランス）" も問題になっています．つまり，できない人の方が一般的なので，できた場合には，ほめる気持ちを込めて「ありがとう（Thank you/I appreciate...）」と言ってみましょう．

腰椎穿刺
Lumbar Puncture

Track 66

看 ハービーさん，和田医師から説明があったように，これから腰椎穿刺の検査を行います．検査の前にお手洗いに行っておきましょう．	Mr. Harvey, as Dr. Wada told you, we will now perform a lumbar puncture on you. Before we start, please go to the bathroom.
患 はい，わかりました．検査中，家族はここに居てもいいですか？	OK, will do. By the way, during the exam, is it OK for my family to stay with me?
看 申しわけありませんが，ご家族の皆さんは，**待合室でお待ち頂けますか？**(⇨ OP)　終わったらお知らせします．	I'm afraid not. **I recommend that your family have a seat* in the waiting room**. Once we are done, I will be sure to let them know.
家 はい，お願いします．	Yes, please do.
患 準備できました．	OK, I'm ready.
看 では，ベッドに横になって，私の方を向いて下さい．	Alright, please lie down on your side and face me.
患 これでいいですか？	Like this?
看 ええ，そうです．今度はおへそを見るようにあごを引いて，背中を丸めて，膝をかかえましょう．	Yes, that's fine. Next, please look down and try to see your belly button. You should curl your back and hold your knees.
…………	…………
はい，そうです．動かないように少し押さえますが，苦しくないですか？	Yes, that's perfect. To keep you from moving, I am going to hold you still. How are you doing?

---

* "have a seat" は熟語．人数に関係なく，ひとりでも複数でも，席を勧める場合には"have a seat"で OK です．覚えておきましょう．

患	大丈夫です.	I'm OK.
看	和田医師が針を刺す部位を今から消毒します. 少し冷たいですよ.	Now, Dr. Wada is going to sterilize the area of your back where he will puncture you with a needle. It's going to be a little cold.
患	….	(No comment.)
看	次に和田医師が背中に局所麻酔の注射をします. 少しチクッとします.	Next, Dr. Wada is going to give you a local anesthetic. You are going to feel a little sting.
患	….	(No comment.)
看	いよいよ背中に穿刺します. 動かないようにしましょう.	Now he is going to perform the puncture, please hold still.
患	….	(No comment.)
看	髄液を採取しています. もうすぐ終わりますから頑張りましょう.	He is now extracting some spinal fluid. This will be over in a minute. Hang in there!

▶ Optional Vocabulary

腰椎穿刺　lumbar puncture 医,　spinal tap 常

Optional Phrases

◘ 待合室でお待ち頂けますか？　　I recommend that your family have a seat in the waiting room. Please wait in the waiting room. Please have a seat in the waiting room.

Additional Phrases

◘ デイルームでお待ち頂けますか？	Please have a seat in the dayroom. Please wait in the dayroom.	より丁寧 ↑
◘ 廊下でお待ち頂けますか？	Please wait in the hall.	
◘ 食堂でお待ち頂けますか？	Please wait in the cafeteria.	

心 電 図
Electrocardiogram (ECG)

看 スペンサーさん，これから心臓の状態を調べるために心電図をとります．

Ms. Spencer, in order to see the condition of your heart, we are going to do an ECG.

患 初めてなので，どんなものですか？

This is my first time. What's going to happen?

看 ベッドに寝て，胸と手足に電極を付けるだけなので，痛みはありません．

You'll lie down on the bed and I will attach electrodes to your chest, wrists, and ankles. Don't worry; this won't hurt.

患 それは嬉しいわ．

I am glad to hear that!

看 ではまず，腕時計を外して，靴下を脱いで下さい．次に，パジャマのボタンを外して，下着を脱いで仰向けに寝ましょう．

OK, first, take off your watch and remove your socks. Next, please unbutton your pajama top and remove your bra. Now, lie flat on your back.

患 これでいいですか？

Is this OK?

看 はい．寒くはないですか？

Yes. Are you cold at all?

患 ええ，大丈夫です．

No, I'm fine.

148　V. 検　　査

看　緊張していると筋肉が動いて正確な測定ができませんので，深呼吸してリラックスして下さい．

Remember, if you are nervous and you move around, we won't get a true reading. Please try to relax and take deep breaths.

患　(深呼吸する)

(Inhales deeply.)

看　クリームを少し塗ってから，胸に六つの電極を付けます．

Now I am going to apply a little cream and six electrodes to your chest.

患　….

(No comment.)

看　両方の手首と足首にも電極を付けます．力を抜いて楽にしていて下さい．では検査を始めます．

Next, I will apply electrodes to your wrists and ankles. Please relax. OK, let's start the exam.

....

はい，終わりです．電極を外して，クリームを拭き取りましょう．

Alright, we're finished. Let's remove the electrodes and wipe off that cream.

患　結果はいつわかりますか？
(⇨ OP)

When should I know the results?

看　あとで飯田医師からほかの検査結果と一緒に詳しい説明があります．

Later on, Dr. Iida will explain the results of this test with the other exam results in great detail.

Optional Phrases

◘ 結果はいつわかりますか？

When should I know the results?
When will I know the results?
When will I know my results?
When will I know my test results?

付　　　録

付録A： 診察申込書
付録B： 外来問診表
付録C： 入院時の持ち物リスト
付録D： 外出・外泊届
付録E： 胃カメラ検査問診表

付録 A 診察申込書

診 察 申 込 書

　　　　　　　　　　　　　　　　　　　　　年　　月　　日

・氏　　名

・国　　籍
・性　　別　　　　　男　　　　女
・生年月日　　　　　年　　　　月　　　　日（　　　歳）
・住　　所

・電話番号

・職　　業

・健康保険　　　　　加入している　　　　加入していない
・海外旅行者保険　　加入している　　　　加入していない
・健康保険に未加入の場合，全額自己負担になりますがよろしいですか？
　　　　　　　　　　はい　　　　相談したい

Appendix A Patient Information

Patient Information

Month (　　) Day (　　) Year (　　)

· Name (First and Family):

· Nationality:
· Gender: Male or Female
· Date of Birth and Age:
· Current Address:

· Telephone Number:

· Occupation:

· Are you enrolled in the Japanese Health Insurance Plan?

　　　　Yes　　　No

· Are you enrolled in traveler's insurance?

　　　　Yes　　　No

· Do you understand that if you are not enrolled in the Japanese Health Insurance Plan, you will have to pay upfront?

　　　　Yes　　　I would like to consult with someone.

付録 B 外来問診表

外来問診表

　診療を効率よく行い，患者さまにも満足して頂けるように，現在の状態や今までのことについて，事前にお聞きするものです．該当する部分にご記入下さい．

　　　　　　　　　　　　　記 入 日　　　　年　　　月　　　日

・氏　　名

・生年月日　　　　　　年　　　　月　　　　日（　　歳）

・性　　別　　　　　男　　　　女

・国　　籍

・どのような症状で受診されますか？
　　　発熱　　頭痛　　吐気　　嘔吐　　咳　　喉の痛み　　胸痛
　　　腹痛　　腹部膨満感　　下痢　　便秘　　体重減少
　　　腫瘤（しこり）　　めまい　　倦怠感　　その他（　　　　　）

・それはいつごろからですか？

・その症状で他の医療機関を受診したことがありますか？
　　　いいえ
　　　は　い（　　　　　　　　　　　　　　　　　　　　　　　）

・今までにかかった病気があれば ○ で囲んでください．
　　　糖尿病　　高血圧症　　喘息　　腎臓の病気　　心臓の病気
　　　結核　　肝臓の病気　　胃腸の病気　　脳梗塞
　　　甲状腺の病気　　精神疾患　　癌　　その他（　　　　　　）

・上の病気は治りましたか？
　　　いいえ
　　　は　い（　　　　　　　　　　　　　　　　　　　　　　　）

Appendix B Outpatient Questionnaire

Outpatient Questionnaire

In order for us to provide the best treatment possible and to see to it that you are fully satisfied, we appreciate your answering some questions about your current condition and your previous medical history. Please fill in the appropriate blanks.

Today's date: Month　　　Day　　　Year

- Name (first, middle, last):

- Date of birth and age (M/D/Y):
- Gender: male or female
- Nationality:

- What symptoms are you experiencing?
    fever　　headache　　nausea　　vomiting　　cough
    sore throat　　chest pain　　stomach pain
    bloating　　diarrhea　　constipation
    rapid weight loss　　lump　　dizziness　　fatigue
    Other (　　　　　　　　　　　　　　　　　　　　)

- When did your symptom(s) start?

- Have you been to another physician about your symptom(s)?
    No
    Yes (Explain:　　　　　　　　　　　　　　　　　　)

- Please circle the illnesses you have had before:
    diabetes　　high blood pressure　　asthma
    kidney disease　　heart disease　　tuberuclosis
    liver disease　　stomach or intestinal ailments　　stroke
    thyroid disease　　mental illness　　cancer
    Other (　　　　　　　　　　　　　　　　　　　　)

- Do you still suffer from any of the above?
    No
    Yes (Explain:　　　　　　　　　　　　　　　　　　)

付録 B（つづき）

- 手術を受けたことがありますか？
    - いいえ
    - は　い（   　　　　　　　　　）

- 現在服用している薬がありますか？
    - いいえ
    - は　い（   　　　　　　　　　）

- 薬や食べ物にアレルギーはありますか？
    - いいえ
    - は　い（   　　　　　　　　　）

- タバコを吸いますか，あるいは吸っていたことがありますか？
    - いいえ
    - は　い　　　本/日
    - 禁煙後　　　年

- お酒を飲みますか？
    - いいえ
    - は　い（種類と量は？   　　　　　　　　　）

- 1カ月以内に海外へ行ったことがありますか？（来日後1カ月以内ですか？）
    - いいえ
    - は　い（国名　　　　　帰国・来日時期　　　　　）

- 女性のみ：
    - 現在妊娠中ですか？　　いいえ　　はい　　わからない
    - 授乳中ですか？　　　　いいえ　　はい

以下は看護師が測定をお手伝いします
- 身　長　　　　cm　　　　体　重　　　　kg
- 血　圧　　　　mmHg　　　脈　　　　　　/分
- 体　温　　　　℃

Appendix B (Continued)

- Have you ever had surgery?
    No
    Yes (Explain:)
- Are you on any medications?
    No
    Yes (Explain:)
- Do you have any drug or food allergies?
    No
    Yes (Explain:)
- Do you smoke or have ever smoked?
    No
    Yes
        How many packs a day?
        Quit smoking since_____
- Do you drink?
    No
    Yes
        Type of drink and how much?
- Have you been abroad in the past month?
  (Have you been in Japan less than a month?)
    No
    Yes
        Country name/date of entry (   )
- For female patients only:
    Are you pregnant?
        No   Yes   Possibly.
    Are you breastfeeding?
        No   Yes
- A nurse will help you with the following measurements:
    Height: cm   Weight: kg
    Blood pressure: mmHg   Pulse: /minute
    Temperature:

付録 C 入院時の持ち物リスト

入院時の持ち物リスト: 以下をお持ち下さい.

- □ 保険証（日本の）
- □ 診察券
- □ 印　鑑
- □ 小　銭
- □ 筆記用具
- □ 寝巻またはパジャマ（有料ですが病院でもご用意できます）
- □ ガウン（羽織るもの）
- □ 下着類
- □ 普段着（外出や外泊用）
- □ スリッパ（すべりにくく，履きなれたもの）
- □ 食事用具（はし・スプーン・ストローなど）
- □ 湯飲みまたはマグカップ
- □ 洗面器
- □ 歯ブラシ
- □ 歯磨き粉
- □ プラスチックのコップ
- □ 石けん，ボディーソープ
- □ シャンプーなど
- □ 身体を洗うスポンジ
- □ ひげそり
- □ く　し
- □ 普段お使いの基礎化粧品
- □ バスタオル2枚
- □ フェイスタオル3枚
- □ ティッシュペーパー
- □ 洗濯物を入れる袋
- □ くず入れ用のレジ袋など
- □ 普段内服している薬（あれば）
- □ 普段お使いの方は：眼鏡・補聴器・入歯用品

- ■ 寝具（布団，枕，毛布）は病院で用意いたします．
- ■ 病院は大勢の方が出入りします．盗難防止のため，貴重品や多額の現金はお持ちにならないで下さい．
- ■ 万一，紛失・盗難にあわれても病院は責任を負えません．
- ■ 院内にはキャッシュコーナーがありますので，ご利用下さい．
- ■ 収納スペースが限られておりますので，必要最低限のものをお持ち下さい．

Appendix C Checklist of Items for Hospital Admission

Checklist of Items for Hospital Admission

- ☐ health insurance card (Japanese)
- ☐ patient ID card
- ☐ hanko (personal seal)
- ☐ small change
- ☐ writing materials
- ☐ pajamas
- ☐ robe
- ☐ underwear
- ☐ street clothes
- ☐ slippers (with good traction)
- ☐ eating utensils (chopsticks, spoon, straw, etc)
- ☐ coffee mug
- ☐ wash bowl
- ☐ tooth brush
- ☐ tooth paste
- ☐ plastic cup
- ☐ soap
- ☐ shampoo
- ☐ wash cloth
- ☐ shaving set
- ☐ comb
- ☐ lotions and face creams
- ☐ two bath towels
- ☐ three hand towels
- ☐ box of kleenex*
- ☐ a bag for your laundry
- ☐ plastic bag for garbage
- ☐ prescription medications (if necessary)
- ☐ if necessary: glasses, hearing aid, dentures

- ■ Bedding will be provided by the hospital.
- ■ As the hospital is open to the public, please refrain from bringing cash or valuables with you.
- ■ The hospital bears no responsibility for lost or stolen items.
- ■ For your convenience, there is an ATM in the hospital.
- ■ Due to limited storage space, please refrain from bringing unnecessary items with you.

* 商品名が代名詞として使われています.

付録 D　外出・外泊届

外 出・外 泊 届

　　　　　　　　　届け日　　　年　　　月　　　日

届け者氏名 _____

患者氏名 _____

　下記により

　　　　　□外 出　　　□外 泊

させたいと思いますので，よろしくお願いします．

外出の場合　　月　　日　　曜日　　時　　分から　　時　　分まで
外泊の場合　　月　　日　　曜日　　時　　分から
　　　　　　　月　　日　　曜日　　時まで

行 き 先

目　　　的

同行者氏名

連絡先・電話番号

Appendix D Permission to Leave/Stay Out Overnight

Permission to Leave/Stay Out Overnight

Submission Date   Year   Month   Day

Name of requesting person _____

Name of patient _____

Seeks to
☐ leave   or   ☐ stay overnight outside of the hospital.

For short leave: Month   Date   Day
    from   hour   min   to   hour   min.

For overnight stay:
    Month   Date   Day   from   hour   to
    Month   Date   Day   hour   min.

Destination

Purpose

Name of Accompanying Person

Address/Phone number

付録 E　胃カメラ検査問診表

胃カメラ検査問診表

氏　名＿＿＿＿＿＿＿＿＿＿＿＿＿＿＿＿＿＿＿＿＿＿＿＿

検査予約日時　　　　　年　　　　月　　　　日
来院時間

＊検査をより安全に行うために，以下の質問にお答えください．

・胃カメラを受けるのは何回目ですか？
　　初めて　　　　（　　　　）回目

・2回目以上の方：喉の麻酔で気分が悪くなったことがありますか？
　　いいえ　　　　は　い

・初めての方：薬や注射，歯の麻酔で気分が悪くなったことがありますか？
　　いいえ　　　　は　い

・心臓の病気がありますか？
　　いいえ
　　は　い（高血圧・不整脈・狭心症・心筋梗塞・その他　　　　）

・血液の流れをよくする薬を飲んでいますか？
　　いいえ
　　は　い（薬剤名　　　　　　　　　　　　　　　　　　　　　）

・眼科で，緑内障や眼圧が高いと言われたことがありますか？
　　いいえ　　　　は　い

・糖尿病または甲状腺の病気がありますか？
　　いいえ　　　　は　い

・男性の方：前立腺肥大症（尿の出が悪い）ですか？
　　いいえ　　　　は　い

・女性の方：現在，妊娠していますか？
　　いいえ　　　　は　い

・取外し可能な入歯はありますか？
　　いいえ　　　　は　い

Appendix E Gastroscopy Patient Questionnaire

Gastroscopy Patient Questionnaire

Full Name (First, Last):

Exam Date (M/D/Y):
Hospital Arrival Time:

- How many times have you undergone a gastroscopy?
  First time?
  　　(　　) times

- If this is your second time (or more): Did the anesthesia you receive make you feel sick?
  　　No　　Yes

- If this is your first time: Have you ever felt sick after receiving anesthesia in a pill or shot form or when going to the dentist?
  　　No　　Yes

- Do you have any heart issues?
  　　No
  　　Yes　(High blood pressure, irregular heartbeat, angina, heart attack, other
  　　　　　　　　　　　　　　　　　　　　　　　　　　　)

- Are you currently taking a blood thinner?
  　　No
  　　Yes　(Medicine name: _____)

- Have you been diagnosed as having glaucoma or high eye pressure?
  　　No　　Yes

- Are you diabetic or have thyroid disease?
  　　No　　Yes

- (For men only) Do you have an enlarged prostate (trouble urinating)?
  　　No　　Yes

- (For women only) Are you pregnant?
  　　No　　Yes

- Do you have dentures or partial dentures?
  　　No　　Yes

索　引

あ　行

赤くなる　redden　40
悪性　malignant　124
あご　chin　138
足　feet（複数）　127 / foot（単数）
　　　　127 / leg　96
足首　ankle　148
頭　head　37
圧迫する　apply pressure　133
アレルギー　allergy　154
安定剤　sedative　110

胃　stomach　112, 143
胃カメラ　gastroscopy　83, 142, 160
胃カメラ検査問診表　gastroscopy patient questionnaire　160
息切れ
　——する　be out of breath　103
行き先　destination　158
医師　doctor 層　15 / physician 医　15
以前に　in the past　132

痛い　sore　126
　それは痛かったことでしょう
　　I am sure that hurt.　39
　　I am sure that was painful.　39
　　I bet that hurt.　39
　　That must have been really painful.　39
痛み　pain　40, 95, 117
痛む　hurt　37, 74, 126, 137, 147
痛みますよね
　　I am sure you're hurting all over.　99
　　I am sure you're in pain.　99
　　I understand you're in pain.　98

1日1回　once a day　90
一日中　all day long　10
胃腸病　stomach or intestinal ailment　152
1階　the first (1st) floor　22, 48
一般食　regular diet　71
入歯　denture　113, 120, 156, 160

うがいする　gargle　110
受付　front desk　43 / reception　26 / reception desk　19
腕　arm　40, 133, 137

＊　この索引では，病名，症状，薬に関する用語のほかに，患者との応対に役立つように，実際の看護現場で使われる表現なども取上げた．

英字新聞　English newspaper　8
　　　／newspaper in English　8
栄養指導　nutritional guidance
　　　　　　　　　　　　92
ATM　automated teller
　　　machine 常　22／
　　　bank machine 常　22／
　　　　　　　cash machine 常　22
延期する　postpone　110
炎症　inflammation　88
エント　discharge　19

嘔吐　vomiting　152
お通じ　bowel movement　74
お腹　abdomen　108, 118
オリエンテーション　orientation
　　　　　　　　　　　　67
終わる
　終わりました
　　I'm done.　41
　　We're finished.　40
　　We're done.　41
　〜はもうすぐ終わります
　　〜 will be over soon.　10
温度　temperature　128

か　行

科　department　16
階
　1 ――　the first floor　22
　2 ――　the second floor　58
　地下1 ――　the first floor of
　　　　the basement　19
海外旅行者保険　traveler's
　　　　　　　insurance　150
会計　cashier's counter　22, 46

外出・外泊届　permission to leave
　　　　／stay out overnight　158
外出許可　permission for brief
　　　　　　　　leave　78
階段　stairwell　69
外来問診表　outpatient
　　　　　　questionnaire　152
加湿器　humidifier　82
貸す
　〜を貸して頂けますか？
　　Can I borrow 〜?　18
風邪　cold
　〜をひく　catch a cold　110
風邪気味　catching a cold　32／
　　　coming down with a cold　32
風邪薬　cold medicine　31
下膳車　cart　72
家族　family
　――以外　people outside the
　　　　　　　　family　24
　ご――の方ですか？
　　Are you a family member?
　　　　　　　　　　　　24
　〜のご――ですか？
　　Are you a member of 〜's
　　　　　　　family?　58
　　Are you a relative of 〜's?　59
　　Are you family?　59
　　Are you related to 〜 ?　59
肩　shoulder　138／upper arm
　　　　　　　　　　　　143
かつら　wig　113
カテーテル　catheter　86, 88
過敏症　allergy 常　133／
　　　sensitivity 医　133
〜過敏症である
　　be allergic to 〜 常　132
　　be sensitive to 〜 医　133
　　have a/an 〜 allergy 常　133
　　have a/an 〜 sensitivity 医　133
カフェテリア　cafeteria　124

索　　引　　165

我慢する
　我慢して下さい
　　Brace yourself.　39
　　Hang in there.　39
髪　hair　138
体　body　141
体の向き　97
カルチ　cancer　19
カルテ　chart(s)　14, 26 / clinical record医　27 / patient file常　27
癌　cancer　152
看護師　nurse常　15 / RN(registered nurse)医　15
看護する　care for　63 / look after　63 / take care of　63
看護暦聴取　nurse interview　80
患者　client医　15 / patient常　15, 115
感染　infection　88
完全静脈栄養(中心静脈栄養)　total parenteral nutrition(TPN)　89
肝臓病　liver disease　152
浣腸　enema　111, 113
頑張りましょう
　　Hang in there.　146

着替え　clothes　67, 89
聞く　hear
　聞こえますか?
　　Can you hear me?　56
傷　incision　108 / wound　37
貴重品　valuables　54, 156
ギプス　cast　19
気分
　――が悪い　feel awful　134 / feel bad　134 / feel funny　134 / feel sick　140, 160 / feel terrible　134

気分(つづき)
　ご――はいかがですか?
　　How are you?　9, 81
　　How are you doing?　81
　　How are you feeling?　81, 122
きまり　regulation　100 / rule　101
気持ち　feeling
　お――はわかります
　　I understand your feelings.　8
救急外来　emergency room　56
救急患者　emergency patient　56
救急車　ambulance　56
狭心症　angina　160
胸痛　chest pain　31, 152
許可　authorization　78 / consent　78 / permission　78
局所麻酔　local anesthesia　111 / regional anesthesia　111
気をつける
　お気をつけて
　　Please be careful.　78
筋肉　muscle　98
　――が弱る　muscle atrophy医　99 / muscle loss常　99
筋肉注射(筋注)　intramuscular injection(IM)　89

具合
　――が悪い　be under the weather　44 / don't feel good　44 / feel bad　44 / feel ill　44 / feel sick　44 / get sick　44
空気マッサージ器　air massager　122
駆血帯　tourniquet　133
薬　drug　154 / medication　46, 154, 156 / medicine　46, 74, 91, 142 / meds　7, 46, 75, 84, 90, 95 / pill　84, 90

薬指　index finger　137
口　mouth　118
首　neck　98
車いす　wheelchair　18, 86, 98
車いす用トイレ　wheelchair accessible toilet　20
クレジットカード　credit card 㕯　22 / "plastic" 㕯（俗）　22
訓練する　practice　117

携帯電話　cell phone　70 / cellular phone　70 / mobile phone　69 / smart phone　70
経腸栄養　enteral nutrition　89
外科　surgery department　20
けがをする　be injured　37
下剤　laxative　110
血圧　blood pressure (BP)　16, 29, 76, 84, 90, 93, 154
　——を計ります
　　We'll check your blood pressure.　30
　　We'll take your blood pressure.　30
血液　blood　137
血液検査　blood test　35, 132
結果　result　148
結核　tuberculosis　152
血管　vessel　86
結婚指輪　wedding band 男　121 / wedding ring 女　120, 121
血栓　blood clot　122
血糖値　blood glucose level　71 / blood sugar level　136
血糖値検査　blood sugar test　136
下痢　diarrhea　152
玄関　entrance
　——脇　by the entrance　18
現金　cash　22, 54, 156

健康診断　check-up 㕯　16 / health screening 医　16 / physical exam 㕯　16
健康保険　health insurance　150
検査　exam　77, 83, 143, 148 / test　35, 56, 116, 124, 132, 140
検査結果　exam result　148 / test result　148
検査室　exam room　77 / examination room　142 / testing room　135
検査用紙　testing sheet　137
倦怠感　fatigue　152

高血圧　high blood pressure　152, 160
公衆電話　pay phone　69
甲状腺の病気　thyroid disease　152, 160
抗生剤　antibiotics　46
声をかける
　声をおかけ下さい
　　Be sure to tell us.　28
　　Please inform us.　28
　　Please let us know～.　27
顧客　customer　144
呼吸する　breathe　117, 143
呼吸方法　breathing technique　117
国籍　nationality　150, 152
腰　waist　138
個室　private room　51
個室料金　private room fee　51
子供の入室禁止　no children allowed　70
困ったこと　complication　106
ゴムバンド　rubber band　138
ころぶ　fall over　37
コンタクトレンズ　contact lenses　114 / contacts　113, 114, 120

さ 行

最小侵襲手術　minimal invasive surgery　107
支える　support　98
刺す　prick　137
寒い　chilly　123 / cold 122, 129, 147 / feel a chill　123
酸素マスク　oxygen mask　127
サンルーム　sunroom　65

次回　next time　43
試験開腹　exploratory surgery　107
時刻　73
自己紹介　self-introduction　62
指示　direction　140
姿勢　position　95, 97
失礼します
　Sorry to bother you.　62
CT検査　CT scan　140
支払い方法　how to pay　22
しばらく　a little longer　77 / for a while　110, 126 / for some time　108
市販薬　medicine from a drugstore　32 / non-prescription medicine　32 / OTC medicine　31, 32 / over-the-counter medicine　32
耳鼻咽喉科　ear, nose, and throat doctor　20
しびれ　numb　127
シャーカステン　display　19
週　week
　——に一度　once a week　67

周手術期　105
住所　address　150
手術　operation 常 111, 126, 128 / procedure 医 111 / surgery 常 106, 108, 111, 113, 115, 117, 122, 124, 126, 152
手術着　operation gown　120 / surgical gown　113
手術後　post-op　117
手術室　operating room 常 113, 114, 120 / operating suite 常 114 / operating theater 医 114 / OR 120, 122, 128 / surgery room 常 114
手術室看護師　OR nurse　115, 124
手術中　mid-operation　124
受診
　——したいのですが
　　Can I see a doctor?　15
　　I insist on seeing a doctor!　15
　　I need to see a doctor.　15
　　I really need to see a doctor!　15
　　I would like to see a doctor.　14
出血　bleeding　133
出身
　ご——はどこですか?
　　Where are you from?　5
術前　pre-op 常 107, 110 / preoperative 医 107
術前オリエンテーション
　preoperative guidance　106
授乳　breastfeeding　154
腫瘍　tumor　124
腫瘤(しこり)　lump　152
準備　preparation　107, 110, 113
　——として　to get prepared　84 / to get ready　84 / to prepare　84

準備する　get ready　123 / prep　123 / prepare　123
紹介状　letter from a doctor　15 / letter from another doctor 常　15 / letter from your doctor 常　15 / letter of introduction 常　14 / referral 医　15 / referral letter 医　15
消化管　gastrointestinal (GI) tract　142
症 状　symptom　31, 152
ほかに何か——はありますか？
　Do you have any other symptoms?　16
　What else is bothering you?　17
　What other symptoms do you have?　17
状 態　condition　147
床頭台　cabinet　67
消毒する　sterilize　133, 146
消毒薬　antiseptic　132, 137 / bactericide 医　133 / cleaner　133 / disinfectant　133
小児科　pediatrics　20
上 部　upper　142
職 業　occupation　150
食 事　diet 医　72, 92 / food 常　72 / meal　72
食事制限
　——を守りましょう
　We need you on a healthy diet.　72
　We need you to stick to a strict diet.　72
　You must be on a prescribed diet.　72
　You need to follow a strict diet.　72
褥 瘡　bedsore 常　96 / decubitus ulcer 医　96 / pressure sore 常　96 / pressure ulcer 常　96

食 堂　cafeteria　147 / dining room　71
食 欲　appetite　76
書 式　form　48
初 診
　——の方ですか？
　Is this your first time here?　27
　Is this your first time to come here?　26
　Is this your first time to come to this department?　27
初診者　first-time patient　14 / new patient　14
処 置　procedure　88
処置室　treatment room　37
処方する　prescribe　46
処方箋　prescription　46
書 類　form　25, 48
心筋梗塞　heart attack　160
寝 具　bedding　54, 101, 156
深呼吸　deep breath　117, 126, 148
診 察　examination　43 / physical examination　34
診察券　patient ID card　14, 19, 26, 43, 156
診察室　examination room　34
診察申込書　patient information　150
侵襲的手術　invasive surgery　107
心 臓　heart　147
腎 臓　kidneys　92
心臓カテーテル　cardiac catheterization 医　87 / heart cath 常　87
心臓カテーテル検査　heart cath exam　86
心臓病　heart disease　152
腎臓病　kidney disease　152
診断書　medical certificate　48

索　引

身長　height　28, 154
　　──は～cm です
　　　You are ~ centimeters tall.　28
　　　Your height is ~ centimeters.　30
心電図　electrocardiogram (ECG)　147
心配
　　～が──である　be anxious about ~　116 / be worried about ~　116
　　ご──ですよね
　　　I am sure you must be worried.　52
　　　I can't imagine how stressful this must be for you.　52
　　　I know how worried you must be.　52
　　　I know how you feel.　52
　　　I know how you must feel.　51
　　ご──なく
　　　Be at ease.　45
　　　Don't worry.　45, 109
　　　Please be at ease.　44
　　　Please don't worry.　45
心配事　concern　103, 116 / worry　104
腎不全　kidney failure　93
深夜　midnight　110
診療科窓口　department reception desk　26

髄液　spinal fluid　146
水分　fluid　81, 85 / liquid　85 / water　85, 141
吸う（息を）　inhale　117, 126, 148
すぐに　on short notice　35
少し　a little　38, 126
　　──したら　after a little while　40 / in a little while　41

頭痛　headache　16, 40, 76, 90, 152
ストレッチャー　stretcher　113, 121
ストロー付きカップ　cup with a built-in straw　108

生検　biopsy　107
清拭　bed bath (BB)　66 / sponge bath　66
正常です
　　This is normal.　30
　　You are healthy.　30
精神疾患　mental illness　152
生年月日　date of birth　150, 152
性別　gender　150, 152
咳　cough　31, 32, 76, 91, 152
　　痰のからむ──　phlegmy cough　81
説明　explanation　26, 106, 128
説明する　explain　46
背中　back　34, 145
洗浄する　clean out 常　37 / cleanse 常　38 / irrigate 医　38
全身麻酔　general anesthesia　110
喘息　asthma　152
洗面器　washbowl　54
前立腺　prostate　160

造影剤　contrast agent 常　141 / contrast dye 常　140 / contrast medium 医　141 / radiopaque dye 医　141
臓器　organ　93
総合案内　general reception desk　14
創処置　wound treatment　37
挿入する（管を）　intubate　126

そけい部　groin 男 87 / upper thigh 87
そのとき　at that time 106, 113

た 行

退院　hospital discharge 102
体温　temp 74, 76 / temperature 29, 76, 154
体温計　thermometer 74
大事
　お——にどうぞ
　　Get well soon. 45
　　Have a nice day. 45
　　I hope you feel better soon. 45
　　I hope you get well soon. 45
　　Please take care. 44
　　Take care. 45
体重　weight 28, 154
　——は～kg です
　　You are ～ kilograms. 29
　　You are ～ kilos. 30
　　You weigh ～ kilograms. 30
　　Your weight is ～ kilograms. 30
体重計　scale 29
体重減少　rapid weight loss 152
倒れる
　突然——　black out 常 56 / experience syncope 医 57 / faint 常 56 / lose consciousness 医 57 / pass out 常 57 / suddenly fall 常 57
たくさん　a lot of 137
出す(書類などを)
　～をお出し下さい
　　Please give me ～. 27
　　Please hand me ～. 27
　　Please show me ～. 26

ただれ　rash 132
立ちくらみ　faint 91
食べ物　food 154
痰　phlegm 常 81 / sputum 医 82
段差　bump 37
胆石　gallstone 106
タンパク質　protein 93

地下1階　the first floor of the basement 19
注意　direction 144 / instruction 142
注射　injection 医 41 / shot 常 40, 89, 143
注射箇所(部位)　injection site 医 41
注射する　give a shot 常 41 / give an injection 医 41
中心静脈栄養　intravenous hyperalimentation (IVH) 89
腸　gastrointestinal tract 111 / GI tract 111 / intestine 112
超音波検査室　ultrasound room 19
調子が悪い(機械の)
　broken 男 75 / busted 常 75 / not working properly 75 / on the fritz 常 75
治療　treatment 88
治療食　special diet 71
鎮静剤　anesthetic 121 / sedative 113

使う　use
　～をお使い下さい
　　Fell free to use ～. 18
　　Please use ～. 18
　　You can use ～. 18

索 引

都合
　ご——はいかがですか？
　　What date and time is convenient for you?　43
　　What day and time is convenient for you?　45
　　When can you make it?　45
　　When will be good for you?　45
伝える　inform　125 / let one know　124 / tell　125
勤め先　place of work　49 / workplace　49
爪　fingernail　110

定期的　from time to time　122
T字帯　loincloth　108
低侵襲手術　minimally invasive surgery　107
デイルーム　dayroom　147
手首　wrist　148
手伝う
　お手伝いが必要ですか？
　　Do you need a hand?　18
　　Do you need any assistance?　18
　　Do you need any help?　18
手続き　procedure　49
テープ　bandage　38
電解質　electrolyte　93
電極　electrode　147
電源　electric outlet　69
点滴　intravenous injection 医　89 / IV 常　88, 122, 140
電話番号　phone number　44, 158 / telephone number　150
　——の発音の仕方　44

トイレ　bathroom 常　113, 120, 135, 145 / ladies room 女　135 / little boy's room 幼　135 / little girl's room 幼　135 / men's room 男　135 / restroom　135 / toilet 常　65, 135
同意書　consent form　142
同行者　accompanying person　158
どうなさいましたか？
　Can I help(you)?　17
　How can I be of assistance?　17
　How can I be of help?　8, 16, 17
　May I help(you)?　17
　What's wrong?　7, 17
糖尿病　diabetes　152
糖尿病の　diabetic　71, 160
床ずれ　bedsore 常　96 / decubitus ulcer 常　96 / pressure sore 常　96 / pressure ulcer 常　96
土足厳禁　no shoes allowed　70
トレイ　tray　7

な　行

内科　internal medicine　16, 20
内視鏡　endoscopy　142
内視鏡的手術　endoscopic operation　107 / endoscopic surgery　107
ナースコール　nurse call　67, 82
ナースステーション　nurses' station　65, 69, 78
名前　name
　お——を言って頂けますか？
　　Can I have your name?　134
　　May I confirm your name?　134
　　May I have your name?　134
　　Please tell me your name.　134

名前(つづき)
お——を教えて下さい
Can you tell me your name? 56
Say your name. 57
What's your name? 57

2階 the second floor 58
荷物 belonging 34 / stuff 54
入院 admission 62 / hospital admission 156 / hospitalization 49
入院受付 admissions desk 49
入院する be admitted 医 35, 76 / be hospitalized 常 35, 76 / check into the hospital 35
入院料金 hospitalization fee
～は——に含まれております
～ is/are all included in your hospitalization fees. 55
～ is/are covered by your hospitalization fees. 55
～ is/are covered by your insurance. 55
入浴する bathe 110
尿 number one 常 135 / pee 幼 135 / pee pee 幼 135 / urine 医 92, 135
尿器(しびん) urinal 医 87 / urine bottle 常 87
尿検査 urine test 135
妊娠している pregnant 154, 160

脱ぐ remove 147 / take off 30
～を脱いで下さい
Please remove ～. 30
Please take off ～. 30
塗る(クリームを) apply 148

熱 fever 32 / temperature 31
ネブライザー nebulizer 81
寝巻 night gown 54 / pajamas 54 / sleep wear 54
眠い sleepy 95, 122
眠る fall asleep 121
年号 73

脳梗塞 stroke 152
濃度 concentration 88
喉 throat 126
——の痛み sore throat 152
ノートパソコン laptop computer 69
飲む(薬を) take
何かお薬を飲みましたか?
Did you take any drugs? 32
Did you take any medicine? 32

は 行

肺炎 pneumonia 35, 117
拝見
——してもよろしいですか?
May I have a look? 7
——する
Let me have a look. 74
配膳車 cart 71
排尿 go number one 常 135 / go pee 幼 135 / go pee pee 幼 135 / urinate 医 135
入る
入ってもよろしいですか?
May I come in? 62
剝がす remove 40 / take off 41
吐き気 nausea 74, 152
——がある feel nauseous 126
吐く(息を) exhale 118

索　引

初めて　first time　51, 147
　〜は——ですか?
　　Is this your first time 〜 ?　14
はじめまして
　Nice to meet you.　124
外す　remove　120, 138, 142 /
　　　　　　　take off　147
発熱　fever　152
鼻　nose　118, 143
針　needle　146
腫れ　puffiness　41 / swelling　41
腫れる　swell　40
絆創膏　bandage　40, 133
反対側　opposite direction　96

日帰り手術　ambulatory
　surgery 医　107 /
　day surgery 常　107 /
　　　　　　outpatient basis 常　107
皮下注射　subcutaneous injection
　　　　　　　　　　　(SC)　89
膝　knee　37, 145
非常口　emergency exit　65
非侵襲的手術　non invasive
　　　　　　　surgery　107
ビタミンD　vitamin D　93
日付　73
必要であれば
　if necessary　19 / if need be　18
微熱　little fever　74 /
　mild fever 常　29 /
　　　　　　　slight fever 常　29
病気　illness　152
病棟　floor　50 / hospital floor
　65 / patient care unit　50 / unit
　50 / ward　49
昼間　daytime　44
疲労感　fatigue　40, 41 /
　tiredness　41 / to be worn out
　　　　　41 / weariness　41

頻度の表し方　112

拭き取る　wipe off　148
副作用　adverse effect(s)　91 /
　adverse reaction(s)　91 / side-
　effect(s)　91 / side effect(s)
　　　　　　　　　　　　40, 91
腹痛　stomach pain　152
腹部膨満感　bloating　152
服薬指導　medication instructions
　　　　　　　　　　　　　　90
不整脈　irregular heartbeat　160
風呂　bath　65
　——に入る　take a bath　40
プロテクター　protector　138
分数の読み方　136

ベッド　bed
　——の端　edge of the bed　98
ペット持込み禁止　no pets
　　　　　　　　　allowed　70
便秘　constipation　152

保険　insurance　51
保険会社　insurance company　48
保険証　health insurance card
　　　　　　　　　　　14, 156
補聴器　hearing aid　156
骨　bone　93
ほめ言葉　119
ホルモン　hormone　93

ま　行

まくる(袖を)　roll up　133
麻酔　anesthesia　106, 113, 160
麻酔剤　anesthetic　84, 128, 143,
　　　　　　　　　　　　　146

待合室　waiting room　22, 145
待つ　wait
　お待たせしました
　　Thank you (so much) for waiting.　28, 30
　　Thanks for waiting.　30
　お待ち頂けますか？
　　Can you wait 〜?　25
　　Do you mind waiting 〜?　24
　　I am sorry, but can you wait 〜?　25
　　Would you mind waiting 〜?　25
　　You have to wait 〜.　25
　少しお待ち下さい
　　Please have a seat.　17
　　Please wait a minute.　17
　　Please wait a moment.　17
　　Please wait a sec.　17
　　Please wait a second.　17
末梢静脈栄養　peripheral parenteral nutrition (PPN)　89
窓側　next to the window　64 / window-side　64

耳鳴り　buzzing in the ear 常　16 / ringing in my ear 常　16 / tinnitus 医　16
脈　pulse　29, 74, 76, 154

向きを変えて下さい
　　Please turn around.　34
胸　chest　37, 122, 138, 147
無料　free　51

目　eye
　――を開けて下さい
　　Can you look at me?　57

目を開けて下さい（つづき）
　　Can you open your eyes?　56
　　Open your eyes.　57
迷惑
　〜に――をかけないようにお願いします
　　Don't bother 〜.　70
　　Please be sure not to bother 〜.　70
　　Please don't be a nuisance to 〜.　70
　　Please don't bother 〜.　70
眼鏡　glasses　113, 142, 156
めまい　dizziness　91, 152
　――がする　feel dizzy 常　16 / dizzy 常　16, 98 / vertigo 医　16
面会受付　visitor's counter　24
面会時間　visiting hours　24
面会簿　visitor's log　24
面接　interview　80
面倒
　ご――ですが…
　　I know I am asking a lot, but…　52
　　I know it's a pain, but….　52
　　I understand it's irritating, but…　52
　　I understand it's troublesome, but…　52

申込書　application form　48
申しわけありませんが
　　I am afraid, …　26
　　I am sorry, …　27
　　I am sorry but as you can see, …　27
目的　purpose　158
もむ　rub　121, 133
問診　brief interview　31
問診表　questionnaire　26, 142

や　行

休む　rest　96
薬局　pharmacy　46

夕食　dinner　110
輸液　transfusion 医　89
輸液ポンプ　infusion pump　74
輸血　blood transfusion 医　89
湯たんぽ　hot water bottle　82
指　finger　133, 137

洋式　western style　65
様子
　少し──を見ましょう
　　I'll make a note of it.　75, 77
　　I will check again later.　75
　　We will keep an eye on it/you.　75
　　We will see how things go.　75
腰椎穿刺　lumbar puncture 医　145 / spinal tap 常　146
よかったです　That's good.　29
4人部屋　four (patients) to a room　52 / four-patient room　52 / four-person room　52
予防注射　immunization shot　40, 132
予約　appointment　43, 142
予約票　appointment card　19, 43

ら　行

楽にしていて下さい
　Just relax.　36
　Please don't worry　36

楽にしていて下さい（つづき）
　Please make yourself comfortable.　36
　Please try to relax.　34

理解
　～は──できましたか？
　　Could you follow ～？　36
　　Did you get ～？　36
　　Did you understand ～？　36
　　Were you able to follow ～？　36
　　Were you able to understand ～？　36
リハビリテーション　rehabilitation　95, 98
良性　benign　125 / non-malignant　125
緑内障　glaucoma　160
リラックスする　relax　148

レントゲン　X-ray　77, 138
レントゲン検査室　X-ray room　35, 138
連絡
　病院に──して下さい
　　Contact the hospital.　40
　　Feel free to contact the hospital.　41
　　Give us a call.　41

廊下　hall　65, 147

わ

脇の下　under your arm　29
和式　Japanese style　65

第1版 第1刷 2011年2月15日 発行
第3刷 2019年1月15日 発行

看護師のための
英会話ハンドブック

Ⓒ 2011

著　者　　上　鶴　重　美
　　　　　Eric　M. Skier

発行者　　小　澤　美奈子

発　行　株式会社 東京化学同人
東京都文京区千石3-36-7（〒112-0011）
電話 03-3946-5311・FAX 03-3946-5317
URL: http://www.tkd-pbl.com/

印刷・製本　株式会社 アイワード

ISBN 978-4-8079-0731-1
Printed in Japan
無断転載および複製物(コピー, 電子データなど)の無断配布, 配信を禁じます.

薬学生・薬剤師のための
英会話ハンドブック
第2版

原 博・Eric M. Skier・渡辺朋子 著
新書判 2色刷 256ページ 本体2700円+税

音声データ
ダウンロード
サービス付

薬局や病院で薬剤師が，英語圏の患者に対応するときに役立つ実践的な英会話集．OTC薬の販売，受診勧奨，服薬指導，病棟での治療薬の説明など実際の場面に沿った会話例を豊富に収載．ネイティブスピーカーにより収録された全ダイアログの音声データダウンロードサービス付．

薬学生のための**実践英語**

Eric M. Skier・上鶴重美 著
A5判 96ページ 本体1600円+税
CD付

海外研修への参加，英語での学会発表，就職活動などを始めようとしている薬学部の学生向け教科書．口頭や書面での自己紹介の仕方や面接の受け方，メールや履歴書の書き方，プレゼンテーションのコツなどを幅広く紹介する．

郵便はがき

1128790

125

（受取人）
東京都文京区　千石三1-三六1-七

東京化学同人
看護師のための
英会話ハンドブック　係

料金受取人払郵便

小石川局
承　認

8658

差出有効期間
2021年1月
31日まで

〈キリトリ線〉

「看護師のための英会話ハンドブック」に対する
ご意見をおきかせ下さい

看護師のための
英会話ハンドブック

CD 無料引換え申込葉書

・この葉書1枚につきCD1枚を無料でお送り致します．
・下記にお届け先をご記入のうえ，ご投函下さい．
 （そのまま宛名ラベルとして使用させていただきますので，
 ご住所，お名前を楽書でお書き下さい．他の目的には使用
 しません．万一，表面の料金受取人払の有効期間が過ぎていても，料金は
 当方で負担しますのでそのままご利用下さい．）

〈キリトリ線〉

お届け先
〒

ふりがな
ご芳名

様

電　話

勤務先または学校名

単位の換算表（概算）

身　長[†1]

インチ 〔in〕	フィート/インチ 〔ft/in〕	センチ 〔cm〕
46	3 ft 10 in	115
48	4 0	120
50	4 2	125
52	4 4	130
54	4 6	135
56	4 8	140
58	4 10	145
60	5 0	150
62	5 2	155
64	5 4	160
66	5 6	165
68	5 8	170
70	5 10	175
72	6 0	180
74	6 2	185
76	6 4	190

[†1] 1 ft = 30 cm = 12 in,　1 in = 2.5 cm
　　1 cm = 0.4 in = 0.033 ft